Praise for *Because I'm Not Myself, You See*

'Blistering, beautiful, true: Ariane Beeston exposes the myth of new motherhood as a loved-up dream, revealing how the transition to motherhood is sometimes a perilous one, and love for our babies hard-won. Written with a careful brilliance, it makes a case against secrecy and shame, and advocates for honesty, empathy and love.'
—Susan Johnson, author of *From Where I Fell*
and *Aphrodite's Breath*

'This is a beautifully written, raw and important memoir for anyone who has had a baby. Even if you have not struggled with mental health, the context in which all women in Australia mother is fundamental to understanding so many of the issues we have in our society. Ariane writes so honestly, and holds your hand through her struggles and coming out the other side.'
—Daisy Turnbull

'A memoir like no other ... Beeston manages the rare trick of making complex ideas about mental health and its absence comprehensible to lay readers, as well as making this dark time sing with mordant humour on the page.'
—Geordie Williamson, *The Australian*

'Ariane Beeston's honesty, poetry and wisdom will save lives. This book is a vital contribution to a reality of some motherhoods that is so often overlooked in favour of stigma, shame and misunderstanding. With insights like Beeston's, we stand some chance of shifting the conversation around psychosis and recovery.'
—Anna Spargo-Ryan, author of *A Kind of Magic*

T0342794

'This book is smart, important and unflinching. It stands on the cliff and dives off with one brave breath. Ariane Beeston gives voice to what many women experience at varying levels and in doing so will make others feel less alone.'
—Megan Rogers, author of *The Heart Is a Star*

'Both riveting and informative, this is an unflinching look at what it is like from inside postpartum psychosis. Writing with insight and compassion, Beeston weaves in research on perinatal mental health and society's attitudes to motherhood alongside her own (impossible) determination to be the perfect mother.'
—Anne Buist, Professor of Women's Mental Health, University of Melbourne, and co-author with Graeme Simsion of *The Glass House*

'This is a polished, sophisticated memoir. And I see myself on those pages, as a mother, a psychologist and a writer. Ariane has given so much of herself in this story and yet showed so much restraint.'
—Lauren Keegan, perinatal psychologist and author of *All the Bees in the Hollows*

'This book is for anyone who has had a baby and felt not quite right, or for family and friends desperate to help but not knowing how. It is also for the health professionals who care for them … This is brave and vulnerable and raw and a much-needed story of hope.'
—Kylie Orr, author of *Someone Else's Child*

'The writing is so evocative, her voice both true and unique. I've laughed and cried, and been shocked by how poorly perinatal health is understood in this country … I feel this book deep in my bones, especially the dark humour.'
—Carly-Jay Metcalfe, author of *Breath*

Because I'm Not Myself, You See

A memoir
of motherhood,
madness &
coming back
from the
brink

You See

Black Inc.

**Ariane
Beeston**

Published by Black Inc.,
an imprint of Schwartz Books Pty Ltd
Wurundjeri Country
22–24 Northumberland Street
Collingwood VIC 3066, Australia
enquiries@blackincbooks.com
www.blackincbooks.com

9781760644505 (paperback)
9781743823569 (ebook)

 A catalogue record for this
book is available from the
National Library of Australia

Cover design by Alissa Dinallo
Text design and typesetting by Aira Pimping
Cover images: Falling woman: Bruce Christianson / Unsplash; Flowers:
Happypatterndesign / Shutterstock
Author photograph by Jodie Mcbride

Excerpt of 'At Last the New Arriving' by Gabrielle Calvocoressi © Gabrielle
Calvocoressi, Persea Books 2009, reproduced by permission of the author; excerpt of 'The
Glass Essay' by Anne Carson, from *Glass, Irony, and God*, copyright © 1995 Anne Carson,
reprinted by permission of New Directions Publishing Corp.; excerpt of *The Crying Book*
by Heather Christle © 2019 Heather Christle, reprinted with the permission of The
Permissions Company LLC on behalf of Catapult Books; excerpt of 'When Absence
Becomes a Form of Presence' by Chelsea Dingman, first published in *The Missouri
Review*, 46.4 (Winter 2023), reproduced by permission of the author; 'Why Bother?' by
Sean Thomas Dougherty, from *The Second O of Sorrow*, BOA Editions 2018, reproduced
by permission of the author; excerpt of 'Mother Who Gave Me Life' © Gwen Harwood,
reprinted by permission of the estate of Gwen Harwood; excerpt of 'How All Things
Are Managed' by Elizabeth Lyons, from *The Blessing of Dark Water* © 2017 Elizabeth
Lyons, reprinted with the permission of The Permissions Company LLC on behalf of
Alice James Books, alicejamesbooks.org; excerpt of 'How Becoming a Mother Is Like
Space Travel' by Catherine Pierce, from *Danger Days*, Saturnalia Books 2020,
reproduced by permission of the author; excerpt of 'Parachute' by Maggie Smith, from
Good Bones © 2017 Maggie Smith, reproduced by permission of Tupelo Press.

Printed in Australia by McPherson's Printing Group.

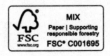

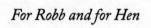

For Robb and for Hen

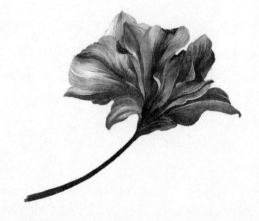

'I can't explain myself, *I'm afraid, sir,'*
said Alice, *'because I'm not myself, you see.'*

LEWIS CARROLL,
ALICE'S ADVENTURES IN WONDERLAND

Here,
I'll begin. As though alive

is not the opposite
      of post-

partum

CHELSEA DINGMAN,
'WHEN ABSENCE BECOMES A FORM OF PRESENCE'

Author's Note

While this is a work of non-fiction, it relies on my memory and interpretations of events. Some names and identifying details have been changed to protect privacy, and some characters are composites for this reason, too.

I have chosen to refer to 'mothers' and 'women' throughout the book for the sake of simplicity and to reflect my own experience, but it's important to acknowledge that not all mothers are women.

The information in this book is based on my experience and research and is not intended as medical advice.

Please go gently as you read. At the back, you will find a list of resources and links to supports and services if you need them for yourself or a loved one.

Contents

Prologue

I'm on my way home from work when my baby turns into a dragon. We are standing at the lights of a busy intersection, waiting to cross the road. The dragon in my pram glares, wiggles its toes. There's a teething rusk in the grip of its hand. This is not the first time it's happened. I've seen dragons before – in the cot, the swings, the highchair. But this one is angry and fierce and red. This dragon is different.

The woman standing next to us smiles at him, leans in to take a closer look. I snap the lid of the pram down and angle the wheels away from her. I must protect my baby from prying eyes. It's hard to know who to trust.

I turn off the main road, pushing the pram along the narrow backstreets. There's a squeal from under the hood, a squeal that settles somewhere in my spine.

When I lift the lid back up, the dragon is gone. My baby, Henry, beams at me, all cheeks and blue eyes.

'Nearly home, buddy,' I tell him. My feet ache in the high heels I wore to the office. It's my third week back at the Department of Community Services after maternity leave. I do not know who

I am anymore or where I have gone, but I can still dress the part.

It's dark now and cold – a clear July night. The stars peek through one by one. When I look down, I can see that my hands are attached to me, but they're no longer mine. I inspect them like a scientist – they're at the end of my arms, my rings are all there. But they don't belong to me.

I call my psychiatrist, Dr Q. The hands still work. She picks up straight away. I've never called her between sessions before.

'I don't think my hands are mine anymore,' I tell her. 'I don't think they're mine.'

'How scary,' she says. 'Where are you, Ariane? Is Henry with you?'

'Yes,' I say. 'But he's a dragon again. We're on our way back from day care.'

'Where's Robb?'

'He's away. For work. LA maybe? Or Singapore? I think he's in LA.' I keep pushing the pram, placing one wobbly heel in front of the other.

Henry points at the neighbour's cat. His squeal again – the way it unravels me.

'I don't know how to explain it,' I say. 'But I just don't feel right.'

'I know,' Dr Q says. And I know she does.

'I'm so tired.'

'You're doing so well,' Dr Q says. 'I'm going to stay with you, okay? Until you get home. Just keep walking.'

I want to curl up in her voice and sleep and sleep and sleep.

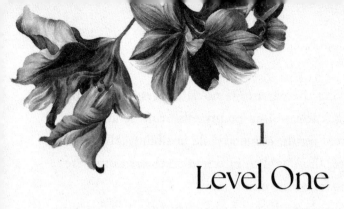

1
Level One

'Respect the delicate ecology of your delusions.'
TONY KUSHNER, *ANGELS IN AMERICA*

The report from the NSW Department of Community Services (DoCS) helpline is a Level One, which means we need to respond to it within twenty-four hours. They're the most serious cases, the most severe instances of abuse and neglect. Sometimes they're high profile and reported in the media: child deaths, murder-suicide or a shaken baby. They're the ones you don't forget.

At times, crisis calls come in from the helpline. Two of us will drop the casework we had planned, to respond to this new information about a child at risk. I come to learn that these calls are most common late on a Friday, as mandatory reporters from schools or childcare centres phone through their concerns before the weekend. There's a predictability about the end-of-week chaos.

We go through these helpline reports with our manager, Megan, and analyse any previous documentation about the families to identify possible patterns. We discuss who we should speak to and what questions we need to ask to see what risks might be present. We put child seats in the government vehicles and head into the field to interview, gather information and make an assessment about a particular case. Sometimes that means bringing a child into care, serving the parents 'removal' papers and driving away. We'll come back to an often-empty office and scramble to find a foster placement for the stunned child or siblings, then pull together – quickly yet thoroughly – information to present to the Children's Court the following day.

During my first week on the job, I accompanied my colleague Rachel as she delivered subpoenas for one of her court cases. It seemed absurd, like something out of a movie – delivering yellow envelopes to a day care and two medical centres while we chatted about our boyfriends and weekend plans. But, as I quickly discovered, that was the nature of the job.

And it's hard. We survive on black humour, coffee, unnatural levels of adrenaline and far too much alcohol on the rare Friday nights we're not out on a Level One. But oh, how I love it. I wanted a job that was meaningful, where I could help others. I am full of naive optimism that that's what child protection caseworkers do – help children and their families. And, in most instances, keep them together.

Today's Level One is allocated to my colleague Clare and me. There's always a primary and a secondary worker when we go out into the field – one to interview, one to take notes – two for safety. Clare has just come back to Australia after working in the London child protection system for two years. She's loud, freckled and hilarious. I'm in good hands with her.

Before we head out, Megan takes us through the report in her office. Her long blonde hair is in a ponytail and she's wearing sensible 'social worker shoes'. Megan is meticulous and unflappable, known for making tough decisions not everyone agrees with.

I joined her child protection team not long after a child death. I missed the immediate aftermath – the investigations, the enquiry by the ombudsman – but we can all feel the impact. The team's practice has been forever changed. One of the many systemic failures identified in the case was not sighting the child, something we now do without fail whenever we visit a family.

'Right. Declan is four months old,' Megan says, scrolling through the report on her screen. Her desk is covered in cream departmental files. 'He's currently in hospital with a cold and severe nappy rash.' Megan clicks on a record about a phone call she made earlier to hospital staff. 'The paediatrician says the rash isn't due to neglect. It got worse after mum tried to treat it with steroid cream, prescribed by her GP. His cold is getting better, too.' She pauses. 'Declan was admitted overnight, so mum – Maggie – and dad – Ben – left baby and went up to the pub on the corner. They had a few drinks and came back to the hospital around ten p.m. While in Declan's room, they had an argument, during which dad allegedly pushed mum against the wall and accidentally bumped Declan's cot. They made so much noise that staff called the police and told them both to leave.'

'Any history?' I ask.

'No DoCS history,' Megan says, 'but police have been to the home a few times for verbal disputes – generally alcohol-related. They were before Declan was born, though. Nothing over the past few months. But we've obviously got concerns for his physical safety, considering Declan is only four months old.'

I remember a line from my training: *The best predictor of future behaviour is past behaviour.*

'Okay,' says Clare. 'What's the plan?'

We decide to interview the paediatrician and hospital staff who saw Declan's parents fighting. We'll also speak to the police and then go to Declan's parents' apartment. When we have more information, we'll consult with Megan to determine the outcome. For now, Declan is safe in hospital. But he'll be ready for discharge soon, so we'll need to make a decision – fast.

It's eleven a.m. by the time Clare and I drive away from the office. It's warm but the sky is threatening rain. I sip the takeaway coffee I grabbed from the café next door and try to eat half a sandwich. It's going to be a long day.

The paediatrician at the children's hospital is busy and matter-of-fact. He confirms that Declan's rash isn't due to neglect and that medically he'll be ready for discharge the following day. 'I'm sorry, I don't know anything else. But you can speak to the social worker.' He looks at his watch and apologises again before disappearing down the corridor.

'They were both very drunk,' the social worker says when we find her in her office. 'Ben pushed Maggie in their room, and she bumped the crib and started screaming at him. That's when staff called the police. Mum says dad has schizoaffective disorder, which is mostly well managed but she's worried he isn't taking his medication. He has another child from a previous relationship, but he hasn't seen her for about four years.' She pauses and checks her notes. 'Dad hasn't been here much, but mum's hardly left Declan's side.'

'And there's an AVO now?' I ask.

'Actually, yes,' the social worker says. 'The police have taken an interim one out. I'll find the number they left. Would you like to see Declan before you go?'

'Yes, please,' Clare says.

Always sight the child.

We follow the social worker down the ward, past rows of closed doors and tired parents. 'Let me know if there's anything else you need from me,' she says, knocking on the door to Declan's room. Inside, there's a nurse hovering over his crib. 'DoCS are here,' the social worker says. 'They just need to see Declan.'

'Of course. Come on in.'

Clare and I peer into the crib.

'He's doing much better this afternoon,' the nurse tells us. 'Isn't he lovely?'

And he is – tiny with dark hair and the sweetest little face, wrinkled with sleep.

'Have you had much to do with the parents?' Clare asks.

'I'm only just back from leave,' the nurse says. 'Haven't even met them.'

'Okay,' Clare says. 'Thank you.'

On our way back to the car, we stop for another coffee. Clare takes a call from the office – one of the parents on her caseload has shown up to their contact visit on the wrong afternoon and has been yelling abuse at Sue, the admin person who took the call.

'I swear I confirmed it on Monday,' Clare says to Sue. She pauses. 'Shit. Maybe I didn't.' She gets in the car and puts her seatbelt on. 'Can you please tell Leanne I'll call her when I'm back in the office? I'll ask if we can arrange another visit. I'm really sorry, Sue.'

'You okay?' I ask Clare, as she hangs up with a sigh.

'Yeah,' she says. 'I think I may have fucked up, though. I told Leanne I'd confirm this week's visit but it must have slipped my mind.'

We're both quiet as she drives out of the hospital car park. My own to-do list keeps me awake and I don't have half as many cases as Clare does.

'Want me to call Megan?' I say.

'Yeah, go for it.'

When Megan picks up, we talk her through what we've learnt about the case: mum and dad both have problems with alcohol misuse and possibly drugs; dad has schizoaffective disorder and might not be medicated; there's a history of family violence, mostly verbal although possibly escalating. There's no family support nearby and no services are currently involved with the parents.

'Right,' says Megan. She pauses for a moment, processing. 'Declan's very young. We need more time to assess what's going on. I'm not comfortable with him going home. Can you get the paperwork ready, please?'

The three of us are silent, considering what this means logistically. Does it sound cold if I admit that the emotion usually comes later? Sometimes it's at home that evening, as the adrenaline quietens and the exhaustion hits. Often it's weeks or months later – during an interview with distraught parents or a difficult day at court. For now, though, there's a task list we must work through – and emotions only slow us down.

Because Declan is in hospital, removing him from his parents is called an assumption rather than a removal (not that this makes any difference at all to the parents whose child is being taken from their care). When he's ready to be discharged, Declan will be brought into statutory care and placed with family members, if they can be found and are considered safe, or approved foster carers, while the case goes to the Children's Court. This can take as long as a year – often longer.

We're not sure how Declan's parents will react, so Megan advises that we take the police with us to the house. We organise for cops from the local station to meet us there and I pull the paperwork from our 'response kit'.

I have only been at the Community Services Centre for about six months, but already I've been involved in taking numerous children into care: a little boy we 'assumed' from his primary school classroom; sisters we took to an aunt's house straight after they'd disclosed being physically assaulted; a boy whose mother relinquished care in a refuge. We've been yelled at, spat at, lunged at. I've been called a cunt. I've worried about being followed home in the dark after work.

Outside the apartment, we wait for the police to arrive. It's three p.m. by now and my head throbs. This part doesn't get any easier and my palms are sweaty in my lap. I wonder if I'm really cut out for this work. Is anyone?

When the cops appear, I slide the assumption papers into my notebook and follow them inside. Maggie is the only one home. She is quiet and subdued as we explain that Declan is now in departmental care. We take her through what's ahead – a contact schedule, a foster placement, help to get her into rehab. I scribble notes down as Clare speaks – this 'interview' will be used as evidence.

It's not until we tell Maggie she won't be able to visit Declan in the hospital that she begins to cry. Contact visits need to be supervised and tend to begin once interim court orders are in place. I hand her a tissue, then another, suddenly conscious of being in her home, her space, her life.

'Is there anyone in your family who might be able to look after Declan?' I ask Maggie. 'Your parents? Or a sibling? An aunt?'

'My mum's overseas,' Maggie says. 'On a cruise. She went on a big trip with her friends. To celebrate her retirement. She'll come back, though. I'm sure she'll come back.'

'Okay,' I tell her. 'Do you know where she is now? Can I please have her phone number?'

As the sun sets, we drive to the children's hospital to update staff about Declan's care and give them copies of the paperwork. The social worker we met earlier has already left for the day and the one on duty knows almost nothing about the case. While Clare explains the assumption paperwork, I text my boyfriend, Robb, to tell him I'll be home late again. We've just moved into a house in Redfern and the place is still full of boxes.

Back at the office, we sit on the floor next to Megan's desk and eat McDonald's. There's rarely time for a formal debrief so it often happens here, on the carpet. While the cleaners move efficiently through the building, we process what's happened and discuss what will come next. Initiating court proceedings sets in motion an array of tasks and deadlines. The day after we remove or assume a child into care, we must file an affidavit for the Children's Court. We have a few hours before Declan is discharged to try to locate family or line up a foster carer. Once we've filed the paperwork, we'll need to set up a contact schedule between Declan and his parents, supervised in one of the tiny rooms in the Community Services Centre and often facilitated by an external agency of young workers who are usually social work students. For a baby as young as Declan, it's normally three one-hour visits per week.

Megan allocates the case to me, adding Declan's name to the whiteboard that dominates a wall in her office before placing mine next to it. He's now the second baby I have on my caseload, along with a two-month-old boy. There are older children, too: Sam, a thirteen-year-old boy in residential care, and four siblings – eleven-year-old Timothy, nine-year-old Jessica, six-year-old Dani and three-year-old Brayden. Depending on our level of experience and the complexity of the matter, we're supposed to have between five and ten cases at any one time – but it's often more.

In a few months I'll have a third baby to look after – Jayde, whose parents police believe are involved in a Sydney drug syndicate. We remove eleven-month-old Jayde in an inner-city police station one Tuesday afternoon. It's another Level One with no prior family history. My colleague Sally and I spend the day interviewing the parents separately and speaking to police about their concerns. The parents give wildly different versions of the night they were arrested, and the father appears drug affected. He sits slumped against the wall of the interview room the police have given us to use for the day.

Later, as Sally holds the little girl, her father – who we later find out was coming down from ice – lunges to attack me. Police appear from everywhere, tackling him to the ground with a thud I'll hear for months, years, to come. He's handcuffed and taken away.

A police officer, a man not much older than Sally and me, picks up a folder and walks past us. 'How can you just take her?' he says. 'This is bullshit. Absolute bullshit.'

I look at Sally, who raises an eyebrow and places a hand on her hip. Sally's almost six feet tall, fiercely intelligent and an excellent caseworker – someone I admire. My hands are shaking and I can feel my face redden.

'I'm really sorry about that,' one of his colleagues says as we get our bags. 'He just had a baby. Last week.'

'Can you please tell me his name?' Sally asks the officer.

'It's Bowen,' he says hesitantly. 'Officer Rick Bowen. But as I said, he just had a baby.'

'Thank you.' Sally scribbles something in her notebook and gestures towards me. 'Let's go.'

Nappy bag over my shoulder and my heart still thrumming, we take Jayde back to the car, where there's a parking ticket waiting for us.

'Of course there is,' Sally says, laughing as she puts the little girl in the worn government car seat. 'Of course there fucking is.'

The police officer who has accompanied us, in case the couple are still in the area, frowns. 'Sorry,' he says. 'Can't help you with that one.'

Sally grabs it, puts it in her folder. Jayde cries all the way back to the office.

I both get used to, and never really get used to, the rhythm of these days.

◇

I fell into child protection work by accident. My honours degree in psychology was useless without the additional two years of study required to be a registered psychologist. Unlike social work, there are no practical aspects of an undergraduate psychology degree (with the exception, perhaps, of conditioning rats to press bars for sucrose). But I was tired of full-time studying and – more importantly – of having no money. I decided to get a job and worry about the extra two years later.

During the final years of my degree, I volunteered as a Lifeline counsellor in Sydney's Northern Beaches. I did a Tuesday afternoon shift each fortnight and an overnight shift once every few months, fuelled by terrible instant coffee that made my heart beat too fast. And while on some shifts it seemed I answered more sex calls than real calls, the training was thorough and the clinical experience was sound. There were mothers I referred to the PANDA (Perinatal Anxiety and Depression Australia) helpline, women with screaming babies I could hear in the background. I was twenty years old and had no reference point for what they were going through, but I knew how to sit with someone in distress – something you can't learn from a textbook.

After I graduated, I applied for a job at Kids Helpline, which was based in Brisbane, not far from where Robb, my on-again-off-again boyfriend, grew up. Our relationship was new and tumultuous – Robb had just come out of a difficult break-up and wasn't ready for 'anything serious', and I wasn't sure I had the patience to wait around until he was.

'Well, I don't believe in monogamy anyway,' I told him, three beers deep at a pub in Pyrmont. 'I don't want to be tied down. I want kids. I really want kids. But I want to do it my way.'

'And what way is that?' he asked with a smile.

'I haven't figured that part out yet.'

We had met in a job interview in a high-rise co-working space in the Sydney CBD. Robb was tall with dark curly hair and kind blue eyes. At the time, he was the community manager for a virtual world and chat room for teenagers, and was looking to employ education and psychology students as online moderators. I was in the third year of my degree, making smoothies at a food court Boost Juice. His job proposition sounded infinitely better than making Strawberry Squeezes and wheatgrass shots for jaded corporates.

I got the job, but not everyone agreed I was suited to the role. 'An online what?' said my brothers, Evan and Huw, when I told them. Robb had called to offer me the position and to invite me into the office for training. 'You can hardly turn the computer on.' (I told them to be quiet then asked them to please show me how because I had a new boss to impress.)

Because the job was completely remote, with four-hour shifts at home around the clock, our friendship developed over AIM and ICQ chats. Our relationship came about a year later when Robb had moved into a more senior role and I was doing my honours in psychology. Robb was funny and intelligent and charming, but it was his calmness I was most drawn to. There was a gentleness about him that settled the churn of my stomach, a feeling that intensified as graduation loomed and I started looking for a full-time job. *Ah fuck*, I remember thinking one afternoon, my books spread around me as I studied for my final stats exams. *I think I'm in love.*

As is often the case when it comes to love, the timing was nothing short of inconvenient. 'I just think I need to be single for a bit,' Robb told me one night. 'Or at least, you know, keep this casual. Isn't that what you wanted, anyway?'

But I no longer knew what I wanted.

When I told Robb that I was considering moving to his hometown, we decided to travel to Brisbane together so I could attend an information day at Kids Helpline and have a look around the city.

Robb's parents lived in Mount Cotton, in the city's south-east. His father was a full-time carer for Robb's younger sister Milly, who had a profound intellectual disability. Physically, Milly resembled a young woman; developmentally, she functioned at around the level of an eighteen-month-old.

I didn't fall in love with Brisbane, but I did fall in love with Robb and with his family. Within weeks, we were living together in a tiny one-bedroom apartment on King Street in Newtown. I was only twenty-one but by then I knew I'd met my person. And so, I declined the interview for Kids Helpline and instead applied for the DoCS helpline in New South Wales. The helpline caseworker role was in many ways the perfect in-between job while I figured out what I wanted to do next. The interview process was intense – a typing test, a panel interview and a role play, which I messed up spectacularly, treating it more like a Lifeline call than a mandatory reporter making a risk-of-harm report. Despite my subpar performance, I got the job. The department was pretty desperate for workers.

The helpline, sprawled across three levels of a building in Sydney's West, felt like a cross between a counselling service and a call centre. It operated 24/7 and had a crisis response team (CRT), which headed out on urgent reports that came in during the night. On the phones, we took calls from mandatory reporters:

14

police, childcare workers, schoolteachers and hospital staff as well as members of the public. Many related to Family Court matters, with one parent calling to report against the other – 'He took them to the beach without sunscreen', 'She sent them to school without lunch'. After each call, we would consult with our team leader about its urgency. There were several factors we considered with each case: the vulnerability of the children, any history on file, the opportunity for harm and any protective factors. Cases were assigned a Level One, a Level Two (response required within seventy-two hours) or a Level Three (within ten days). Reports from open cases – those with an allocated caseworker out in the field – were sent through to the local office managing it, while others were closed at the helpline with no further action taken.

During peak periods – lunchtime and between about six p.m. and ten p.m. – the floor manager would stroll between cubicles, looking up at the digital board that flashed red as wait times increased, eyeing anyone not on the phone. I came to dread the moments when, having just hung up and still scrambling to piece together whatever narrative I'd just been told, I'd feel a tap on my shoulder and hear: 'Do you mind just picking up that one, please?' It was the floor manager's job to keep wait times down, and their bosses' job to answer to the minister if they got too high. It was my job to hear and process and carry and triage whatever trauma lay at the other end of the line.

The work ranged from repetitive and straightforward to gutting. I answered calls about serious non-accidental injuries and allegations of sexual abuse that we sent through to the Joint Investigative Response Teams (JIRT), made up of police and DoCS. Despite the subject matter, the professional callers were easier to handle than those from the community. During one shift, a man whose child had been removed by the local office yelled at me for almost half an hour. No matter how many times I gave the standard line, 'I'm sorry, I've made a note of your concerns and I'll send them through to the caseworker,' I just couldn't end the call. We circled for a while, covering the same ground as he simultaneously fired accusations at me while acknowledging that it wasn't my fault. I remember this call because it's the only one where, defeated, the tears came before I hung up. My voice didn't waver, but I cried silently while typing up his concerns. I was coming off a week of night shifts, and the sleep deprivation made me more fragile, less resilient.

A colleague alerted my team leader, Molly, who wrote 'Want to put him through to me?' on a piece of a paper. Molly was warm and bubbly but extremely protective of her team.

I shook my head. 'Alright,' I said to the caller, 'I am sending this through to the local office now. They'll be in touch. Take care.'

'What happened?' Molly asked as I hung up. 'Are you okay?'

'Yeah,' I lied. 'Just a tough one. His kids were removed a month ago and he says no one at the local office is returning his calls. I'll send it through to them.' I took my headset off and locked my computer. 'Going to the bathroom. I'll be back in a sec.'

It happened. Not often, but it happened. We cried or vented or laughed, even when it wasn't funny, and then we moved on to the next call.

During the helpline's two weeks of training, a far-too-perky presenter claimed, 'One of the best parts of this job is that you don't take any work home. Once you've logged off for your shift, that's it!'

Except it wasn't like that at all for me. I may never have literally taken files home to work on at night or over the weekend, but the calls, the stories, followed me wherever I went. When I found myself answering calls in my sleep, not able to switch off even in my dreams, I started thinking it might be time for a change – and to finish my last two years of study.

I applied for and was offered a position as a field caseworker at a Sydney community service centre. According to the Psychology Board, I could count some of the hours as placement towards my psychologist registration too. No more long train commutes and maybe a little more work–life balance with a nine-to-five schedule that wouldn't mess with my sleep cycle and moods as much.

Well, that's what I thought.

∽

While I had hoped that Declan would be restored to his mother's care, it's looking less and less likely. Maggie has been in and out of rehab – at least four centres by now – and Ben has stopped answering his phone. For now, though, Declan is safe with his grandmother Kim, who returned from her overseas trip immediately after Declan first went into foster care. Declan is healthy and thriving, and the department recommends that Kim be granted parental responsibility for him. This would make her Declan's legal guardian until he turns eighteen.

Kim is in her early sixties, recently retired and ready to travel the world. She's absolutely enamoured of Declan, but she hadn't anticipated raising him into adulthood. While there was never any question of her stepping in to care for Declan in the short term, she's sad, torn and exhausted.

'I'm so disappointed in you, Ariane,' Kim tells me at court after receiving the department's care plan for Declan. She, too, had hoped Declan would be returned to Maggie. This outcome is not uncommon, or at least it wasn't then – it's considered a way to promote long-term stability for the child and to allow them to develop an attachment to their primary caregiver. But Kim's words pierce; until then, we'd had a good relationship. She had seen me as an ally. Now I am the enemy.

It's a part of the job that I struggle with. I am known for being kind and empathetic, for building good relationships with the parents I work with. When the outcomes aren't what they expect, families see it as even more of a betrayal.

Ben reappears and leaves abusive and often drunk voicemails on my phone, demanding access to his son and calling me names, before phoning back to apologise. But when I finally organise a contact visit for him after months of not seeing Declan, he doesn't show up. I catch the lift downstairs to where the contact worker is waiting with Declan. He smiles at me from his pram – so much bigger than when I last saw him.

'Hello, beautiful boy,' I say, before thanking the worker for waiting. 'I'm so sorry. Ben's not coming. Can you please take Declan back home?'

When I call Ben, it rings out.

Because Maggie is challenging the department's recommendation that Kim have long-term parental responsibility for Declan, we head back to the Children's Court for a hearing. Maggie's team has hired a barrister and I'm terrified of making a mistake or saying the wrong thing. I've only taken the stand twice before, in other cases, and as I read through all the evidence and prepare to be cross-examined, my mouth breaks out in cold sores.

The day before the final hearing, we receive a fax from Maggie's lawyer – Maggie has been discharged from rehab for drinking. Her lawyers agree to Kim having parental responsibility for Declan. The case won't go to a hearing, so I won't be cross-examined after all. We'll need to finalise how much contact Maggie and Ben will have with Declan and what that will involve, but other than that the matter is settled – in the eyes of the court, at least.

When Megan tells me the news, I'm so relieved I could cry. And later, when I get home, I do. I feel gutted for Maggie, for Declan and for Ben. You can't always pinpoint why it happens and I know other colleagues feel the same way about certain families, but some cases get under your skin. This one got under mine. But it also nestled itself in the depths of my brain.

2

And They
Get Removed

'It's bad, isn't it? It's really bad.' I snap a photo of the baby's bare bottom and send it to Robb, who's at work. It's the third photo I've sent that morning and I'm feeling increasingly panicked. I've been rubbing thick white Sudocrem onto the rash for hours but it's still angry and red. It seems to be spreading.

The baby looks up at me with navy-blue eyes I don't recognise. My own eyes are brown – I thought his would be too. Did I take the right one home? How often do babies get mixed at birth?

They're coming for him, I know. The nappy rash is so bad, DoCS are going to take him and everyone will know what a terrible, terrible failure of a mother I am.

They know. They can see it.

I feel as though I might vomit.

I rub more Sudocrem onto the rash and send Robb another photo. 'Does this look bad?' I ask again. 'Is it getting worse?'

'No,' he replies. 'It looks fine to me. But why don't you ask your dad if you're worried? I'm going into another meeting. I'll call you later. I'll be home early.'

I don't ask my father, a GP; instead, I text my mother.

'Oh yes, babies get nappy rash,' my mum says. 'Poor thing. How's he feeding? Did you get much sleep last night?'

'He wakes every forty-five minutes,' I say. 'I can't see straight.'

'I remember those days,' she says. 'I don't think you sleep properly for two years. And then of course you have another.'

Babies get nappy rash, I tell myself. Babies get nappy rash. Babies get nappy rash.

Yeah, and they get removed.

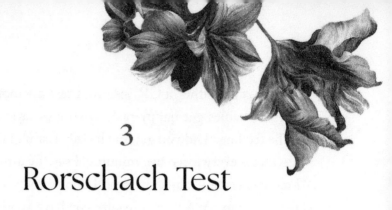

3
Rorschach Test

*'Mothers must perform for me. They must perform
the roles of "encouraging mother", "helpful mother",
"patient mother", "authoritative mother".'*

DR SHARON LAMB, *THE NOT GOOD ENOUGH MOTHER*

My desk phone rings as I'm working out a urine analysis schedule for Matt, the father of fifteen-month-old Jayde. He is subject to a police investigation and Jayde is living in temporary foster care while the case is before the court. Three times a week, Matt must present for supervised urine testing at the local pathology centre. Whether he turns up and what substances are detected will form part of our evidence for the Children's Court.

'I've got Matt on hold,' says Callum, our head of admin.

'Can you put him through to voicemail for me, please?'

I have a dull headache and I can't take being called a cunt again today. I have an unofficial one-cunt-per-day quota.

After eighteen months of shift work at the DoCS helpline and almost two years as a child protection worker in the field, I am completely burnt out. I can't sleep. I can't eat. I'm always cancelling on my friends: 'Sorry! On response and heading out. Can we try again next week?' And I'm forever tired and grumpy and taking it out on Robb. With the long hours at work, including after-hours responses, and needing to collapse in a physical and emotional heap on the weekends, our lives are not as neatly aligned as I'd hoped they'd be when I left the shift work of the helpline.

Around the office, our team is referred to as 'The Removalists' because of the number of children we've brought into care. My colleague and friend, Jo, has a set of nine siblings whose medical, family contact and psychological needs all rest on her shoulders. She is older and more experienced than I am, but even this is a stretch.

We are all far too stretched.

∽

Although I don't smoke, I join Jo for cigarette breaks in the garden downstairs, where we talk about our cases, our days and our lives outside the office. Or what little is left of them.

One afternoon we're standing in the sun, deciphering a text message from Jo's new girlfriend, when she looks at me and leans against the wall.

'Why aren't you eating?'

'What do you mean?'

'Everyone's worried about you.'

'They are?'

'Yep.'

'Have they asked you to say something?'

'Perhaps.'

'Really?'

'Megan said you never eat the sandwiches you buy for lunch.' She looks me up and down. 'And you're getting skinny.'

'Stress,' I tell her. 'It's how my body deals with stress. It just shuts down. And I can't eat. Used to happen at uni, too, whenever I had assessments.'

'Right,' Jo says. 'So, it's not some weird ballerina shit.'

'No,' I say, trying to hide my annoyance. I know Jo has drawn the short straw to interrogate me, but I'm used to checking in on others, and the reverse feels strange. 'I haven't danced for years. It's not that. It's just stress.'

The answer satisfies Jo – we're all stressed. She drinks Tia Maria and Coke most nights; I only eat half my lunch. Her check-in duty done, our chat moves to the two children we removed the day before. At 4.30 p.m. Alice, one of our intake colleagues, called the home of a family whose case had been assigned a Level Three, to be followed up in 'less than ten days'. A little girl answered the phone.

'Hello,' Alice said. 'Who is this?'

'It's Hannah.'

'Hello, Hannah. Is your mum or dad there?'

'No. They went out.'

'Is there anyone else at home with you now?'

'Yes.'

'Who?'

'My brother, Lou.'

'Can you please put him on the phone?'

'He's a baby.'

'Oh. And how old are you, sweetie?'

'I'm four.'

Fuck.

'Who's free?' Megan asked, from the doorway of her office. Jo and I were the only ones not already out in the field. We booked a car, checked it had the correct baby seats and prepared removal paperwork. I phoned the police to ask them to meet us at the apartment block in Surry Hills.

When the cops opened the door to the unit, we found two

kids jumping on a bare mattress on the living room floor. There was a food-stained doona next to it and empty plates and cups. The little boy, who we later found out had only just turned two, had the biggest, cheekiest smile and the dirtiest, heaviest nappy.

Hannah was talkative and friendly. She said her dad had gone out and hadn't come home yet.

'Where's your mum, sweetie?' I asked.

'I don't know,' she said.

'All clear, boss!' yelled one of the cops as he moved from room to room, opening cupboards and wardrobes. I caught Jo's eye and raised an eyebrow – *Yeah, no shit, mate.* The apartment, save for the children, was empty.

While the police talked to the kids, we filled garbage bags with clothing and toys and sheets from their beds. During the forty-five minutes we were in the apartment, there was no sign of either parent. We left the removal paperwork on the kitchen bench.

On the way back to the office, we bought the children Happy Meals. 'Chips or nuggets?' I asked Hannah.

'Nuggets,' she said. 'And Lou wants chips.'

Megan was waiting for us in an empty office when we returned, filling in a care plan for the court.

'Who's this?' she asked, as Hannah ran towards her with a half-eaten chip.

'I'm Hannah,' she said, climbing into Megan's chair. 'Who are you?'

'I'm Megan. Would you like to eat your dinner in here?'

Hannah nodded and while she settled in, I followed Jo back out to our desks.

'I should change Lou,' I told her as she logged back into her computer.

'I will love you forever if you do.'

'You already love me.'

'True.'

Lou smiled up at me while I wrestled with his nappy. Nappy changing wasn't something I had much experience with, so I peeled back the sticky tapes slowly. The nappy wasn't just heavy – it looked as though he hadn't been changed for days. His bottom was red and the smell was overwhelming. I let Lou wriggle away, giggling, while I found a plastic bag. When I carried him back to his sister, they ran around the desks, picking up the phone receivers and pushing the chairs. Neither he nor Hannah cried. Neither of them asked for their parents.

'Indiscriminate attachment,' Jo said later.

'What does that mean?'

'When kids are friendly to anyone who'll pay them attention,' she explains. 'You'll see it a lot with children in care.'

Because the family had no history with the department except for the first report to the helpline, and there were no interviews to type up for the affidavit, we put the paperwork together in record time.

According to a report we received later from the helpline, the children's father returned home at nine p.m. – about three hours after we left – and called to demand his children back. I felt for the caseworker who took the call – it can't have been an easy one to explain, given that the notes we hastily left on the digital file were limited.

In the garden, Jo finishes her cigarette and looks at her watch. 'Right. I guess we should go file, then?' she says.

The paperwork is due at the Children's Court by four p.m. Yesterday, full of nuggets and chips and with Hannah still chatting away, we'd dropped the children at an emergency placement nearby. It's only short term, though, and they'll need to be moved again this evening after we file. The placement team is onto it, ringing through their little black book of emergency foster carers, and we're hoping they find somewhere local. We're both too exhausted to take Hannah and Lou on a long drive.

'Yep, let's go.'

Once the papers are filed in court, they need to be served on both parents. Yes – we do that part, too. And, depending on where the foster placement is, there could still be a long night ahead.

The poet Maggie Smith writes in *You Could Make This Place Beautiful* that memoir can never be a tell-all. Instead, she says, it's a 'tell-mine, and the *mine* keeps changing, because *I* keep changing'. What happens when your memoir is a 'tell-ours' because your story is also your baby's story and your husband's story and for a long time there, when your self disappeared, you were solely defined in relation to them: someone's mother, someone's wife? What happens when your tell-mine is full of gaps? When your tell-mine becomes a tell-ours because so often you simply do not remember what happened? Memory is fallible under the best of conditions, but what about when it's formed in exhaustion and adrenaline, in trauma and madness? We know that mood can affect memory: research shows that depression is linked to poorer memory performance – as is lack of sleep. Which memories can I trust?

Sitting in the sun during week six of Greater Sydney's Covid-19 lockdown, I text Jo, who is isolating in Canberra ahead of his upcoming gender affirmation surgery. Our departmental days are long behind us, but we have remained close friends.

'What do you remember about the children we removed from the apartment block?' I ask. 'The ones who were home alone.'

'Umm, the little girl wasn't sure if I was a boy or a girl?' he writes back.

'Ha!' I reply. 'I remember that.'

I tell Jo that I thought the father had gone looking for drugs, but it's not a clear memory.

'I can't recall what he was doing,' Jo says. 'Did the kids tell us? And I think the mum was overseas?'

'Your memory is terrible,' I say.

'Fucking hopeless,' he texts back. 'I sometimes wonder if too much stuff has happened, and my brain reached overload at some point and every memory replaces an old one.'

I think of the Canadian poet Anne Carson's words:

> *You remember too much,*
> *my mother said to me recently.*
>
> *Why hold onto all that? And I said,*
> *Where can I put it down?*

I am putting it down here, now. I am trying to put it down.

✑

At the helpline, reports of prenatal risk of harm are recorded as 'Unborn' along with the mother's surname: Unborn BROWN, Unborn MILLER, Unborn UNKNOWN. The reasons for a woman being reported during pregnancy are varied: drug or alcohol misuse, concerns about family violence, or already having children in out-of-home care. Some of the babies have birth alerts on their files, which means the hospital needs to notify DoCS the moment they're born. On the child protection team, we are often waiting for these calls.

'The Smith baby is here,' Megan tells me on her way back from the intake desk. 'The helpline just phoned it through. I'm going to let Out-of-Home Care know. Meet me in my office in five?'

I nod and save the case note I've been writing. Unborn SMITH, the child of two Indigenous teenagers, has been listed against my name on Megan's whiteboard for the past few months, and I'm about to find out why.

In the busy maternity ward, the hospital's social worker leads me and my colleague Sam down the corridor. 'They're in this room,' she says, knocking on one of the doors. 'Come and find me when you're leaving. I've got some discharge paperwork for you.'

Bek, who has just turned sixteen, sits on the bed with her newborn son. She has long dark hair, twisted into two messy buns, and is wearing a blue dressing gown. Her mother, Jan, sits beside her, packing nappies into a bag.

'Geez,' Jan says, looking at Sam and me as we walk into the room. 'They start them young in DoCS these days.'

I put the baby capsule down and look at my feet. According to current departmental orders, she's not supposed to be visiting. I let it go, though – today will be difficult enough as it is.

'Hi, Bek,' I say. 'I'm Ariane, Kalen's caseworker. We spoke on the phone last week. And you've met Sam.'

'Hey, Bek.' Sam smiles. 'Congratulations. He's beautiful.'

'Thanks,' she says. 'He is, hey?'

I glance at the clock on the wall. 'Are you almost ready?' I ask Bek. 'We've got a long drive ahead. We told them you'd be there by two.'

'Yep.' Bek doesn't look up as she puts a dummy in Kalen's mouth. 'Give me ten minutes.'

Because Bek is in the care of the department until she turns eighteen, she has her own allocated caseworker, Sam. Before Sam it was Terri and before Terri it was Dan. And that's just over the past two years. Bek has full parental responsibility for Kalen, and I am – we both are – determined to keep it that way. When I watch her with him on the bed and see the pride in her tired eyes, I remember why I'm doing this job – why I'm trying to do this job.

Megan's stipulations are clear and firm: because Bek has no family she can live with safely and is no longer in a foster placement (having been in and out of placements for years), she and Kalen are to stay in a refuge a few hours out of Sydney. The baby's father, who has just turned eighteen, has denied paternity. There are also police reports that he's been physically and emotionally abusive. While staying in a refuge isn't exactly an ideal start to motherhood, I know Bek will be safe there and surrounded by workers who'll help her care for Kalen. And, most importantly, they'll be together.

Downstairs in the car park, I strap Kalen into the capsule while one of the midwives helps Bek out of a wheelchair.

'Now, remember you can call if you need any advice,' the midwife says. 'Alright? Anything at all.'

'I know,' Bek says. 'Thank you.' She groans as she settles beside her son, her bags squished at her feet.

'You okay, Bek?' I ask her, getting into the passenger side.

'Yeah,' she winces, touching her belly. 'Just sore.'

❧

Megan calls while we're sitting in traffic, driving back from the refuge. Getting Bek settled in took longer than we expected and it's peak hour by the time we leave.

'How did Bek go?' Megan asks. I can hear her typing away on her computer, obviously still in the office.

'She was okay, actually,' I say. 'Tired and sore but okay. The staff seem lovely, and she has her own room. She chatted the whole way down – told me she chose the name Kalen because it means "warrior".'

'Oh, that's gorgeous,' Megan says. 'Make sure you write a note about that when you get into the office. Kalen might want to read his file one day. It would be nice for him to see that.'

Two weeks later, it's 9.30 a.m. on New Year's Eve. I hang up the phone and walk into Megan's office. 'That was the refuge,' I tell her, sitting down at her desk. 'They're this close to evicting Bek. She's not following their rules. Turned up after curfew yesterday. She's getting into arguments with other women. And they're worried about the baby – not sure she's coping with him.'

'Is Sam around?'

'I think she's on leave.'

Megan stands up and looks over at the office of the out-of-home-care manager. There's only a skeleton staff on during the holiday period and the out-of-home-care team don't tend to do crisis work.

'I'll see who's here.'

Twenty minutes later, a caseworker I've only seen around the office, Geoff, and I are preparing to drive to the Blue Mountains. It's already midday. Bek doesn't know we're coming – it's an un-announced visit. On the way up, Geoff tells me he has a toddler. He's been an out-of-home-care caseworker for a few years now and prefers the slower pace.

'This reminds me why I'm happy not doing crisis work,' he says, as we crawl along the highway in bumper-to-bumper traffic.

We find Bek standing in the garden, having a cigarette with another woman. She looks surprised when she spots us.

'Hi, Bek,' I say. 'This is my colleague, Geoff. We're here to see you and Kalen.'

'He's with Mandy, one of the staff,' Bek says, defensively. 'I told her I needed a five-minute break. She said she'd watch him.'

'That's okay,' Geoff says. 'We all need breaks. Can we see him, please?'

I'm grateful for Geoff and his knowledge of babies. He asks Bek about Kalen's feeding, how much formula she's giving him, how she measures it out and prepares it, how he's sleeping and where.

I am out of my depth. What do I know about babies?

I tell Bek that Megan and I are trying to get her and Kalen into a special program for young mothers – one that will teach her mothercraft skills and give her more support than she's getting at the refuge.

'They'll want to meet with you first, though,' I tell her. 'Before they decide to take you on. Is that okay?'

'Yep, that's fine.'

It's no secret that of all my clients, I have a soft spot for Bek. She's been let down by the system again and again in ways I will never understand, and I want life to be different for her. I want it to be different for her little boy.

We write a new case plan – Bek agrees to abide by the refuge's rules until we can get her a place in the program. It's almost four p.m. by the time we leave.

'I hope you didn't have any plans tonight,' Geoff says as we get back to the car.

'Not really,' I say, mentally cancelling the New Year's party Robb and I were going to. I know he'll be pissed off that I'm too wrecked to go. He's been looking forward to it, but I'm too tired to do anything much these days.

'You?' I ask Geoff.

'Ha,' Geoff says, turning onto the highway and flicking on the radio. 'Not with a toddler, no.'

Going into the new year I feel a sense of relief. I have a flex day on Monday – three days off. We'll soon get Bek into the program where she and Kalen will be safe and cared for.

How quickly things change.

On Monday, two of my colleagues remove Kalen after Bek breaches several points in the case plan we'd agreed to. She leaves the refuge without telling us where she went, has contact with Kalen's father, is unable to be reached and doesn't take Kalen to hospital when he has trouble breathing – not once, she admits, but twice. It's the hospital staff, when Bek eventually turns up, who make the report to the helpline – a Level One – with concerns for his immediate safety.

My team are told not to tell me until I get into the office. When Megan takes me through what's happened, I burst into tears. I am both relieved I didn't have to remove Kalen and devastated that I wasn't there for Bek.

'It's not your fault, hon,' Megan says. 'I know how hard you tried.' She hands me a copy of the assumption paperwork. 'Can you give the foster carer a call and find out how Kalen went last night? Her name is Lyn. We'll need to consult with an Aboriginal caseworker too. Can you arrange that as soon as you can?'

Because of Bek's extensive history as a child in care, and the amount of casework we've done prior to removing Kalen, there's a lot to piece together for the affidavit, due at court at four p.m.

Geoff drops past my desk with an open bag of jelly snakes, and Jo helps me find key dates in the digital files. I'm still printing off the papers and getting them stamped by a Justice of the Peace at 3.30 p.m.

Megan pokes her head out of her office, where I'm sitting, cross-legged, stapling pages together. 'Can someone drive Ariane to court?' she yells out to the team. I'm newly minted on my red Ps, an absolutely rubbish driver and even worse at parking (particularly when under pressure).

'Yep, I'll grab a car,' Jo says. 'You ready to go?'

'Just.'

We make it to the counter with four minutes to spare.

Back at the office, I call the foster carer Kalen's been placed with in Western Sydney. She's warm and chatty and tells me her children are besotted with him.

'I'll come out and see him next week,' I tell her. 'And I'll be in touch about a contact schedule. It's likely to be three times a week.'

'Yep,' she says. 'I know the drill.'

Nine months later, we will recommend to the Children's Court that the department hold parental responsibility for Kalen until he turns eighteen, the same orders his mum is still subject to. I am, naively perhaps, surprised when Megan tells me about the recommendation – I had still hoped that Kalen would be returned to Bek.

In the end, it's a relatively straightforward case and the final orders are granted soon after we file the papers. Though Kalen is Indigenous, he will remain with the non-Indigenous foster carer with whom he was placed for short-term care. This is despite the care plan I've written for him, which cites the Aboriginal Child and Young Person Placement Principle (ACPP) that, where possible,

Aboriginal children and young people should be placed within their family or community or another Aboriginal community.

Concerns about his 'primary attachment' – the relationship he's formed with his foster carer – have taken precedence.

This is not unusual.

This is still happening. As Professor Megan Davis notes in the 2019 *Family Is Culture* report, the ACPP is poorly implemented and misunderstood. 'The department has lost focus on achieving the fundamental goal of the ACCP: keeping children and young people connected to family, community, culture and country, and recognising community as a strength for children,' she writes. 'This is because the culture of compliance has overwhelmed the other critical skills casework demands: intuition, instinct and judgment.'

As for Bek, she will have contact with her son just six times a year, with additional visits for special occasions.

And the cycle continues.

For us as young caseworkers, the impact of child removal on a parent's mental health wasn't even on our radar. Our workloads were high enough just managing the children in our care and there were always unallocated matters we simply didn't get to. If the parent's mental health problems had been identified prior – for example, Ben's schizoaffective disorder – that was different (and often used against them). But when I think about Maggie and Bek, who were not even six months postpartum when their babies were removed, it's difficult not to feel shame. How could it be that we didn't understand that asking new mothers to jump through often increasingly difficult hoops while recovering from birth, adjusting to motherhood and facing numerous social challenges was setting them up to fail? That having their child taken from them was only going to make their existing mental health issues worse? Years later, I read a Canadian study that describes the experience of having a child removed as a 'living death', as the parents have no control over when or how they can see their child. Not only are they labelled 'bad parents', but the stigma around child removals means they are less likely to ask for or receive social support.

For Indigenous mothers, this traumatic experience is compounded by the continuing intergenerational impacts of the Stolen Generations. Rather than providing genuine support, our system continues to fail Indigenous families – even though we know that Indigenous mothers are more likely to face mental health issues compared to non-Indigenous mothers, both before and after pregnancy. It disproportionately subjects them to surveillance and punitive responses, doing little to address the underlying causes of child protection involvement. We've created a vicious cycle whereby antenatal care isn't considered safe – namely because of the risk that the child will be removed – yet avoiding antenatal care often triggers a risk-of-harm notification by child protection authorities.

I can write here that we all did the best we could at the time, in a broken, racist system. I sometimes even believe that's true when reflecting on my own complicity. We lurched from crisis to crisis, always fearful of making the wrong decision or of missing something important. But that doesn't make it okay. It wasn't okay then and it's not okay now. And while I wish I could say that it's been well over a decade since I worked as a caseworker and the system is now less violent, less intrusive, less punitive, the facts speak for themselves: Aboriginal children are still disproportionately represented in the child protection and out-of-home care system in NSW. The system is still broken; the system is still racist.

∽

Although I later realised that the burnout I felt was from years of hearing and carrying horrific stories of abuse and neglect and trauma, at the time my failure to keep Bek and Kalen together is the moment I realise I can't be a caseworker anymore. I no longer believe I am helping families. How can I, when all I seem to be doing is breaking them apart?

A psychologist position at a DoCS office in Western Sydney comes up, and it isn't just my dream job; it's a step back from frontline child protection work. I want to keep working in child protection – it's in my blood now – but I need to slow down.

Two interviews later, the position, a twelve-month maternity leave cover, is mine. I'm both excited and terrified. I have only twelve months to go until I'm a fully registered psychologist and the position will give me all the training and supervision I need.

However, Megan has been moved into a different role and my new manager won't 'release' me from my caseworker position until I've either closed or handed over all my cases. Four of them, including Kalen's, are still before the Children's Court and will need to be allocated to one of my already stretched colleagues. It's at least a month's worth of work, probably more like six weeks, but I tell them I'll get it done in two. When management continues to push for four more weeks, my team, who recognise how fragile I am, split the remaining cases between them. It's one of the kindest things anyone in the workplace has ever done for me.

I work until midnight every day and come into the office hours before everyone else. I update legal orders, finish case notes, type up interviews I've scribed for my colleagues and complete transfer paperwork. One morning, as I'm getting ready, I bump my hand against the sink while I'm brushing my teeth.

'Fucking piece of SHIT!' I yell at it, hitting the sink back harder.

Robb holds me while I cry into his shirt. 'You're almost there,' he tells me.

On Christmas Eve, a week before I'm due to finish up, Tim, a father who'd recently had his daughter restored to his care, calls me to say he's not sure he can do it. It's the only restoration case I have on my workload and – selfishly, perhaps – one that's kept me going.

'Maybe she'd be better off back in foster care, mate,' Tim says. 'I just don't know if this is going to work out.'

We've worked towards restoration for months and I know, *I know,* it's the best place for his little girl. I swallow my swelling rage, rage that's really my own exhaustion and compassion fatigue and frustration with the system, and I take a deep breath.

'Tell me what's happening, Tim,' I say. 'Is Sammy still having nightmares? How did she go at day care this week?'

Later that night, after awarding myself a Christmas Eve early mark of five p.m., I collapse onto the couch in a room blinking with silver lights. My muscles ache. I've got nothing left.

The trip from Redfern to south-west Sydney takes almost an hour on the train. I meet my new manager downstairs and she takes me up to the office. It's familiar but different, with the same office pods piled high with cream departmental files and faded blue carpet. Later, as I'm setting up my account and logging on to the system, one of the casework managers pokes her head into my office.

'Oh! You're the new *psych*,' she says. 'I saw you earlier down-stairs, but I thought you were a student.'

'I'm older than I look, I promise,' I say, smiling. 'I'm Ariane.'

'Emma. Welcome! We've missed having a psych. I'll tell my team you're here.'

Paul, another psychologist on our district's team, emails to see how I'm settling in. He's the only other psych not on leave and, like me, he's a provisional psychologist working towards full regis-tration. He's also one of the only Indigenous psychologists in the department. I'm not used to working so alone or even having my own office, and the difference is stark.

In the cupboard I find a packet of Rorschach cards, a relic from another time. The famous inkblot test, where a person is asked to describe what they see in the strange artwork, is consid-ered pseudo-scientific and hasn't been used clinically in DoCS for years. The cards are still there, though, tucked alongside the *Diagnostic and Statistical Manual of Mental Disorders* (DSM-IV), IQ tests, child behaviour checklists and bags of puppets. One of the tests, the Bayley Scales of Infant and Toddler Development, is unopened, brand new. As I rifle through the books and read scor-ing manuals, I'm grateful no one can see the size of my grin; I'm exactly where I want to be – my first job as a psychologist.

'Do you have the Rorschach in your cupboard?' I email Paul.

'Yep,' he replies. 'Have you read the manual? It's hilarious.'

◆

In this new job, I'm part of a team covering Metro South-West: Liverpool, Bankstown, Fairfield, Campbelltown and Ingleburn. Although we have our own offices, we meet once a month on a Tuesday for peer support (a formal part of psychologist supervision) and to allocate new referrals. I also meet with a senior psychologist once a week to talk through my work. She signs off on every single consultation I provide. I've never had so much professional support in my life – a far cry from debriefs with cold McDonald's on the office floor.

I no longer fear the 4.30 p.m. crisis phone calls, long nights and cancelled plans. There's time to read and think and reflect on the reports that I'm writing and the cases I'm working on.

My job involves consulting on cases being managed by the child protection teams, the out-of-home-care teams and the early intervention team, as well as working with children in care and their foster carers. I write transition plans for babies moving between foster placements and behaviour management plans for older children. I help write and run a training and support group for out-of-home foster carers. And I learn how to administer and score most of the psychological tests in the cupboard.

I miss the adrenaline of field work at times. I miss working closely with a team and the (rare) days when casework would fall into place. But I don't miss removing children, being yelled at by parents, doing court work or being too stressed to eat or sleep. I don't miss the weight of carrying so much risk, the weight of so much vicarious trauma. And I don't miss the way it was slowly changing me – I was becoming tightly wound, quick to anger, hardened.

During a group training session for foster carers, a colleague introduces the concept of the Circle of Security, a visual 'map' of what's known as attachment theory. Based on decades of research, the Circle of Security helps parents and caregivers meet children's emotional needs, support their exploration of the world and be a safe haven from it, too. The idea is so lovely in its simplicity, so easy to understand, that I print out a copy and put it on my office wall. It guides my practice; I look to it often.

Always be
BIGGER, STRONGER, WISER AND KIND.
Whenever possible
FOLLOW MY CHILD'S LEAD.
Whenever necessary
TAKE CHARGE.

✍

Six months after I begin my role as a departmental psychologist, I'm called back to court to be cross-examined about Jayde, the baby we removed from the police station. Even though I'm no longer the caseworker, my name is on many of the original affidavits and I'm still employed by the department.

The final hearing is set across two days at the Children's Court. To prepare, I read over the original affidavits and try to catch up on what's happened since I handed over the case to Sally. I won't be asked about any of the most recent casework, but I will be asked about some of the earlier decisions we made and, quite possibly, the day we brought her into care.

Now a cheeky, brown-eyed toddler, Jayde has been living in a temporary foster placement with a departmental carer. I learn from Sally's notes that we are recommending the court make long-term orders for Jayde, placing her in foster care until she turns eighteen. Our assessment and the court clinician's report highlight significant concerns about family violence, drug use and illegal activity – and the parents failing to engage with the department in any casework. (The phrase 'failing to engage with the department' makes me wince now. So often it was the department who failed them.)

Restoration is not an option, the notes read. I underline this twice as I prepare to be cross-examined.

On the day of the hearing, up on the stand, I don't make eye contact with Jayde's father, Matt, while I answer questions from his lawyer. It's been a year since the police tackled him to the ground in front of me, but the trauma feels raw.

I've reflected on this case many times over the past decade, but it wasn't until I read *Stranger Care: A Memoir of Loving What Isn't Ours* by Sarah Sentilles that I could articulate what was wrong about how it was managed. In the book, which explores Sentilles' and her husband's attempts to adopt a child in foster care, she explains that in her particular jurisdiction in the United States, the caseworkers who remove a child are not the ones who end up working with the family. I take a photo of the passage below:

> Earlier that week, Grace had called to tell us she would no longer be our social worker. We'd meet our new social worker, whose name was Camilla, at court. 'It's good cop, bad cop,' Grace explained. 'One of us – that's me – takes the child away from the biological mother; the other one of us – that's Camilla – tries to help her get her child back.'

Reading this is a light-bulb moment: I should not have been allocated Jayde's case. What happened in the police station was traumatic. I lay awake many nights wondering, *What if we'd been out in the field alone? What if we hadn't been surrounded by police?* Now I lie awake thinking, *I'd probably react similarly if someone tried to take my child.* And yet I was new and had 'capacity': there was an empty space next to my name on the whiteboard. If you were involved in the removal of a child, you or the secondary caseworker would be given the case to manage. That's just how it worked.

But back to court now. Jayde has her own lawyer too, a harried young man from Legal Aid in an unironed shirt, who asks me questions about why we didn't place her with any of her family and why she remained in a DoCS foster placement. They're standard questions, good questions, and I answer them all confidently – the placement assessments Sally and I completed at the time were rigorous and thorough. Neither the maternal nor paternal grandparents were considered 'safe' options. I am excused from the stand after forty-five minutes.

'Did I do okay?' I whisper to Sally as I slide back into my seat. I can feel the sweat pooling under my arms and take my grey court jacket off.

'Yep. Perfect,' says Sally. 'Also, how do you manage to still look hot on the stand?'

I blush and grin. It's a week before I'm to marry Robb. And now that this court appearance is over, I can relax.

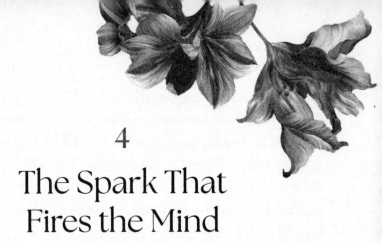

4

The Spark That
Fires the Mind

'When I am sobbing on the bathroom floor,
what does the baby feel?'

HEATHER CHRISTLE, *THE CRYING BOOK*

'So, are we hoping we're pregnant or not?' asks the young woman at the checkout. I'm hedging my bets with a pregnancy test in one hand and a box of tampons in the other, and the question takes me by surprise. But there's a smile across my lips as I head back to the office. My breasts are big and sore and rivered with deep blue veins. I don't need a test to tell me what I already know – we're going to have a baby, a little one of our own.

Robb had wanted to wait, to be married for a while, to be just us. But I want a baby, now, now, now.

I am the eldest of four children who grew up in the chaos and noise and drama of a big family, and I can't imagine not having one or two children of my own. I've planned to have my first baby at the age of twenty-seven – two years after leaving field work – and my second two years later. The maternity leave position I was covering has now become a permanent role and I've been accepted into a Master of Clinical Psychology, which I'll do part-time. I have it all figured out.

Still, it's faster than we expected – much faster. Two couples we are close to have been trying for a baby for over a year, so we assumed it would take us at least a few months, that we would have time to get used to the idea first.

Be careful what you wish for.

We keep my pregnancy secret for the first few weeks, holding it between the two of us. I spin in the kitchen, still light on my toes, my centre of gravity not yet tilted forwards. The excitement is a current – a constant tingling, even as the fatigue sets in, and because of it, too. I imagine the baby's heart beating inside me, its tiny throb.

The worry appears around eight weeks. It wasn't there at all – and then it's there, always. I worry that our baby has a neural tube defect, a condition known as anencephaly. I google, scrolling through page after page of results. 'Neural tube defects are birth defects of the brain, spine, or spinal cord. They happen in the first month of pregnancy, often before a woman even knows that she is pregnant.'

Often before a woman even knows that she is pregnant.

Where did this fear come from? The ferocity of it seizes my thoughts, makes it difficult to concentrate on anything else. I google between case consults at work, google, scroll, google, scroll, click, read, read again.

I tell no one of this worry, the deep gnawing anxiety. I do not even name it, because I am pregnant – delighted, blessed. Instead, I read journal articles, calculate how much folate I may or may not have consumed before I fell pregnant. I was not starving myself before our wedding but I did drop weight accidentally in the lead-up. Have I failed my baby, already?

Often before a woman even knows that she is pregnant.

'Read, learn, work it up, go to the literature,' writes Joan Didion in *The Year of Magical Thinking*. 'Information [is] control.'

Because I believe the damage is done, I am resigned to the inevitable news. I am certain we will be told at our twenty-week scan – the anatomical ultrasound where they check the spine and the heart and the brain – and I gird myself for the force of it. I don't buy any baby magazines or baby clothes. I don't write lists of names or look at prams. I do not allow myself to become attached.

Each morning I wake dry-retching and vomiting, crouching over the toilet bowl or lying on the cold tiles until the nausea passes. Sometimes, it lasts all day. The phrase 'morning sickness' feels like a cruel joke I am not in on. By thirteen weeks, contrary to all the stories I've heard and all the blogs I've read, the vomiting still hasn't passed.

Morning sickness is a good sign! say the baby forums. *Eat crackers! Ginger! Hang in there, mama!*

'Can you see the spine?' I ask the ultrasound technician when she completes the nuchal translucency scan. I am lying on the bed, dressed in my grey work pants, trying to make out the grainy images on the screen.

'Oh no,' she says, handing me a paper towel to mop up the gel. 'Too early.'

I carry white hospital vomit bags on my commute to south-west Sydney when the symptoms seem to be at their worst, and often vomit in the bathrooms at work. One morning I don't quite make it and vomit all over the stairs at Liverpool Station. The shame is hot in my cheeks. I run out of meetings to vomit, I phone in sick again and again. It becomes harder and harder to do my job.

During the second trimester, I travel with Robb to the US on one of his work trips. We drive from LA to Las Vegas and get fake married in a drive-through at the Little White Wedding Chapel, saying vows we made up on the spot through the sunroof of a hire car.

'Can you make a heart shape on her belly?' asks the photographer, who looks like an off-duty Elvis impersonator, when he learns we're expecting a baby. We laugh because it's *just so cringe*. And we do it anyway.

At Disneyland, the nausea is so bad I lie down on the cool platform as we wait for the train to take us around the theme park.

I do not glow. I am not radiant.

༄

'Looks like some of us have eaten a few too many Easter eggs over the break,' one of my ballet teachers says from the front of the class. I am fifteen years old, dressed in our school's uniform of a navy-blue leotard with pink tights. While he puts the Royal Academy of Dance syllabus in the CD player and finds the music for our next exercise, I suck my stomach in and pull the bottom of my leotard down.

I have just started at a North Shore private school after winning a ballet and dance scholarship. After three years at a public high school, it's a shock – blazers and boaters and navy-blue ribbons, fancy hardcover diaries and chapel in the school hall. I had wanted to do ballet full-time by completing school through distance education and dancing six days a week. My parents, however, were understandably reluctant. And so, this is a compromise: I can stay at school, complete my HSC, while going to dance each morning and most evenings. It is a strange existence. As 'ballet kids' we are always missing classes, always catching up, exempt from sport and camp. I am always rushing, from class to school and back to class.

Along with some of my classmates, I'm selected to perform with the English National Ballet in their Australian tour of *Swan Lake*. Backstage, we watch the swans putting on their headpieces and painting their eyes with dark, intricate lines. We take photos with them and ask them to sign our pointe shoes. We scoop up stray sequins and feathers from the dressing rooms and put them in our ballet bags for safekeeping. I have never been more certain of what I want to do with my life – I want to be a dancer.

There are eisteddfods and competitions and exams. There are medals and high distinctions and honours. And as soon as I hit puberty, there is rejection.

After years of intense ballet training, I am used to my body being scrutinised, critiqued. By now, I know that I am too short, too muscular. I am both too much and not enough. I will never be like my classmate Loren, whose impossibly long legs, tiny torso and bendy feet mean she's already been accepted into the Australian Ballet School as an associate. I am technically as good as she is – stronger, perhaps, and just as hard-working – but I will never have the perfect ballet body. The wall of mirrors reflects everything I am not, six days a week.

When my belly starts to show, my body becomes open to public scrutiny again. Where once I felt the sharp fingernails of my ballet teacher under my belly button and between my shoulder blades, now it's intrusive belly touches, and comments on my shape and size. I am praised for the size of my bump, for 'staying neat', 'compact', for not 'letting yourself go'.

'I can't wait to see you get fat!'

'You actually have boobs!'

'You're going to be one of those women who bounces back straight away.'

'At least all the vomiting will keep your weight down.'

'Your face is so round! You look so different.'

At my first antenatal appointment, my obstetrician – a softly spoken man in chinos and a white shirt – asks me to step on the scales in the corner of his office. He peers down at the number under my bare feet and tells me, matter-of-factly, that I should be around 61 kilograms by the time I deliver. I do the calculation in my mind: it's 12 kilograms over my current weight. The number both intrigues and horrifies me. But with a goal in place, I decide that I will be the perfect pregnant woman – at least with the amount of weight I gain. It's something, one thing, I can control.

Along with the pregnancy app that tells me what size my baby is (a strawberry, a capsicum, a watermelon), I find a pregnancy weight-tracker that plots how much weight I should gain over the next few months, week by week. It's not at all reputable, not at all evidence-based, and yet I look at it almost every day. Pregnancy websites all tell me the same thing: the weight is made up of about 3.5 kilograms of baby, a kilo of amniotic fluid, half a kilo of placenta, a kilo of uterus, 1–2 kilograms of blood, almost a kilo of boob and about 4 kilograms of fat tissue. It's familiar territory, this tracking, monitoring, obsessing. And, for the first time since training for a career in ballet, watching the numbers go up on the scale each week stirs a dormant beast.

I was fifteen (tracking, monitoring, obsessing) the first time I tried to shrink. My body, my 5'1 body, took up too much space in the world I wanted to dance in, and I hadn't yet realised – or didn't yet understand – how cruel and ridiculous and unfair this was. I starved, I binged, I purged. I ran and ran until I gave myself shin splints I never quite recovered from. The morning of my school certificate maths exam, I ate only a handful of jellybeans. Maths was a struggle for me regardless and my head was full of clouds. I looked great in a leotard, though; everyone said so.

'We know what you're doing,' my friend Sarah, a fellow ballerina, told me as the weight was disappearing off my bones. 'Don't be stupid.'

But I am not being stupid, I thought. *I am doing what I need to do, doing what so many other women before me have done.* 'Must see the bones,' American choreographer George Balanchine once told dancer Gelsey Kirkland, whose autobiography, *Dancing on My Grave*, I read while starving myself. 'Eat nothing.'

Eat nothing.

I might not have been the skinniest, but my strength as a dancer *was* my strength: my ability to hold the slower adagio exercises without wobbling or to do a triple pirouette almost without thinking; the height of my grand allegro or the big jumps dancers complete at the end of class. When I starve, my strength disappears – I lose my edge.

> *Starve, binge, purge, run, dance.*
> *Starve, binge, purge, run, dance.*

I am mortified when one afternoon I am pulled from my English class and summoned to the deputy principal's office. He shifts, uncomfortable, while I take a seat at his desk. Someone has told him that they saw me in the local Woolworths buying laxatives.

'Do you need me to make a referral to the school counsellor?' he asks.

I am in a flood of tears because although it wasn't me – laxatives are not a weight-loss method I've even thought to try – someone, *someone*, dobbed me in.

My ballet teacher is concerned that I'm still going to evening classes at the school I've trained at since I was twelve. 'It's not good for your legs,' he tells me. At first, I think he's worried I might get injured. Then I realise it's because he thinks my muscles are too big.

'They like shorter dancers in Germany,' another teacher says during a private lesson. She looks my body up and down and nods. 'Ella got into a school over there and you have much nicer proportions than she does.' What she doesn't say is this: Ella has already returned to Australia after six months, homesick and injured. She's quit dancing completely and is completing Year 12 at TAFE.

I dance my HSC ballet exam (a year early as part of the conditions of my scholarship) on legs that scream and throb, in a body with whom I am at war. I hate it and it hates me.

It's another dancer, a few years older and one I admire, who tells me over coffee that if I continue to starve and binge and purge, I might never be able to have a baby. I haven't yet made the link between fertility and being underweight, and it's a jolt. I know exactly what she means: my period had arrived once, over the summer holidays, then promptly disappeared for a year when I began training again. Even as a teenager, I knew I wanted a baby more than I wanted to be thin enough for ballet. And so, over the next twelve months, I slowly, reluctantly and begrudgingly stop trying to punish my body for a dream and begin to eat.

'I can eat anything I want now,' I told my mother when I decided not to pursue a career in ballet. My heart was shattered but I ignored it, throwing myself into study. I was going to be a psychologist. I was going to write. Old dreams would make way for new ones.

'I wish,' Mum said with a sigh. 'We're short, though. Every kilo shows.'

~

'It took me five or six months to show,' essayist and author Leslie Jamison writes in *The Atlantic* of her pregnancy after an eating disorder. 'Before that, people would say: "You don't look pregnant *at all*!" They meant it as a compliment. The female body is always praised for staying within its boundaries, for making even its sanctioned expansion impossible to detect.'

Sanctioned expansion. We are allowed to grow, but not too much.

On Instagram, I come across a vintage Barbie-like doll, the Mommy-to-Be, released in 1992. 'She is more than a toy,' the ad says. 'She provides a natural way for your child to learn while playing. Remove her "pregnant tummy" – and there's her baby. Lift out the baby with its moveable arms and legs and now she has a "flat tummy".' Simple as that, eh?

My obstetrician remarks that my stomach is 'unblemished' by pregnancy. Not only have I stayed within the bounds of the number I was given, but I also don't appear to have any stretch marks.

'You're so lucky!' my friend says sarcastically when I share this story. 'People might still find you desirable! You still have value.'

I am a vessel. I am undamaged goods.

~

As my bump grows, I am intrigued by the archaic way doctors still measure it with a tape measure. The fundal height – the distance from the pubic bone to the top of the uterus – seems almost comedic in its simplicity.

Worried that I'm 'measuring small', my obstetrician sends me for an extra scan. But when the sonographers look closely, the baby is just corseted in, held tight by muscle from years of dance. My skin itches under the stretch of him.

'He's a beautiful, healthy boy,' my obstetrician says.

'Is his spine okay?'

'Everything's perfect.'

Presented with objective evidence from the twenty-week scan that he does not have a neural tube defect, my anxiety wanes, folds back in on itself and settles.

In its place is a strange sort of absence of emotion. I feel neither happy nor sad. I have forgotten how to feel anything.

While my lack of excitement about meeting the baby seems odd and out of step with the anticipation of everyone around me, I put it down to fear of the birth itself, a fear that has grown slowly but steadily.

I walk and wait and walk.

∽

'The most prolific cause of insanity of pregnancy is an hereditary predisposition to insanity that exists, and the events of pregnancy acting simply as the spark that fires the mind,' Dr J.W. Palmer wrote in a 1903 address to the Georgia Medical Association.

I was an anxious child, shy. I picked at my thumb constantly. In primary school I was in an accelerated class with boys two years older. During lunchtime some days one of them would touch me inappropriately in the playground when the teachers weren't watching. I didn't understand what he was doing but I knew it was wrong. I picked at my thumb until it bled and scarred. When my period arrived, I was exquisitely sensitive to hormones. My uni diaries were full of the highest highs – 'Ariane, are you on drugs?' my friends would ask. 'Why are you talking so fast?' – and the lowest lows. When I started taking the contraceptive pill, I was so moody and horrible to live with that it almost ended my relationship with Robb.

But I'd never been diagnosed with anything ... so none of that counted, right?

'Was I ever screened during pregnancy?' I ask Robb as I write this chapter. 'For mental health stuff?'

'Not that I recall,' he says. 'But would you have been honest if you were?'

It's a good question.

It is not so easy to be honest about how bad you're feeling – not when you're supposed to be grateful about having a baby.

⟿

At a perinatal conference in Melbourne recently, I meet an academic who tells me about his work with stressed pregnant guinea pigs. He and his team are looking at the impact of stress on the behaviour and brains of their offspring.

'How does one stress a pregnant guinea pig?' I ask him.

'Strobe lights,' he says. 'Guinea pigs get very stressed under strobe lights.'

I am thinking about the guinea pigs now while I look at research into the impact of anxiety and depression on a developing fetus. It's not a topic I find easy to read or write about. There's guilt and fear and regret. Why didn't I say anything at the time? Why did I suffer through it?

I am learning about fetal programming.

I am learning that while we know that maternal mental illness during pregnancy affects a fetus, we don't know exactly why.

I am learning that babies of depressed mothers are exposed

to higher levels of cortisol and that this can lead to adverse neurodevelopmental outcomes, possibly even transmitting psycho-pathology from mother to child.

I am learning that treatment makes a difference – that taking certain medications during pregnancy is safe and can help. That in many cases it is preferable to *not* treating anxiety and depression antenatally.

I am learning to give myself grace.

∽

I'm pregnant at the same time as supermodel Miranda Kerr, singer Pink and actress Natalie Portman. I have never been particularly interested in celebrity lives, but I find myself scouring the internet for pictures of them to compare the size of our bumps. 'From *Black Swan* to Baby' reads one headline about Natalie, who had existed on a diet of carrots and almonds to play a ballerina in Darren Aronofsky's film. It's a diet I was once familiar with, too. I watch Natalie win an Oscar for the role. Heavily pregnant in a purple dress, she makes pregnancy look easy, even graceful. But while the comparisons make me sting with jealousy, once I've started it's impossible to stop. I obsessively scan the cesspit that is the *Daily Mail*'s Femail for updates on my pregnant posse. Do I 'wear' my bump as well at Natalie? Do I look as fit as Pink?

Miranda is the first of us to give birth, five months ahead of Pink, Natalie and me. While our bumps continue to grow, Miranda returns to modelling – and the media switches to fetish-ising her flat post-baby stomach. 'Cherubic supermodel Miranda Kerr is officially back to work after giving birth to son Flynn in early January and has been snapped looking ridiculously stretch-mark-free in a bikini while shooting for Victoria's Secret in

Malibu,' *Pedestrian* gushes in an article headlined 'Top 5 Post-Baby Body Bounce-Backs'.

Heavily pregnant, I buy a postpartum Belly Bandit online. It promises to 'tighten and shrink' my post-baby tummy and lists Jessica Alba – number four on *Pedestrian*'s list – under its celebrity testimonials. (She'll later sue the company – and win – for using her likeness without permission. Sorry, Jess, it sucked me in too, so to speak.) I haven't even given birth and I am already worried about my own 'body comeback'. What kind of fuckery is that?

'It was easy to call my doctor absurd when she chided me for gaining five pounds in a month (rather than four!) and harder to admit that I'd honestly felt shamed by her in that moment,' Leslie Jamison writes. 'It was harder to admit the part of me that felt a secret thrill every time a doctor registered concern that I was "measuring small." This pride was something I'd wanted desperately to leave behind.'

I so desperately want to leave it behind too.

Years after my own pregnancy, while on staff at Fairfax Media's *Essential Baby*, I write an article with the kind of working headline designed to generate clicks: 'How My Pregnancy Almost Triggered an Eating Disorder'. It's a heavily sanitised version of events, punctuated with caveats ('Of course, I'd never put my baby's health at risk', 'It wasn't easy, but it was worth it').

I find a stock photo, a pregnant woman standing on a set of scales, and hyperlink all the research sources. Normally I'd send it to my editor, who would publish the piece, pitch it to the masthead (*The Sydney Morning Herald* or *The Age*) and share it to social media. For whatever reason, however, this time I don't; the finished article sits in my drafts folder for years, never published.

Even though I'd written deeply personal articles about mental illness, taking psychiatric medications and spending time on a psych ward, talking about the fact that I'd struggled not to lapse into old, disordered eating habits during pregnancy felt even more taboo.

When you write for an online publication, you learn to anticipate the backlash, the comments, the emails. You weigh up the benefits of sharing your story, the traffic, and the emotional toll it might take. And, when it came to this one, I was not ready to give it to the world.

Many women struggle not only with body image, but also with their *feelings* around their struggle. 'I feel like a bad feminist,' a friend texts during her pregnancy, when she admits finding the weight gain difficult. 'But food and exercise are a way to try and feel in control when my body has been taken away from me.'

Another friend, Lizzie, tells me that it took until her third pregnancy for her to finally ask her obstetrician not to weigh her at each antenatal check-up. 'We agreed that when he *did* weigh me, I'd stand backwards on the scale so I couldn't see the number,' Lizzie says. 'It just made me feel too down about myself.'

Research around body image during pregnancy is mixed and complex. For some, the physical changes have a positive effect on how women feel about their bodies because the focus shifts from appearance to the health of their baby. As one published paper opined, weight gain during pregnancy is seen as more 'socially acceptable' than 'mum bods' postpartum. (Note here too that 'dad bods' are often seen as sexually desirable despite doing absolute none of the work involving in growing a baby, while a mum body is something we need to 'fix'.)

In a recent article on the body image of pregnant women one sentence stands out: 'There was an acceptance of a temporary transgression from the body image ideal.' A *transgression*. Where does one even begin with this? To grow a baby is to transgress from ideal beauty standards. But only temporarily – for once we've birthed it's time to go right back. Is it any wonder I bought a bloody Belly Bandit?

∽

On my due date, I waddle down to the local shopping centre. It's midweek, so Robb and all my friends are at work. My hospital bag is packed and waiting at the door.

'When are you due?' the lady at Dymocks asks, as she processes my never-to-be-read pile.

'Today,' I reply.

She looks horrified. 'Should you be out? Shouldn't you be at home with your feet up?'

'It's okay,' I tell her. 'Even if he comes today, I've heard these things can take time.'

'Well, keep your phone handy,' she suggests, handing me my receipt.

It's a solid tip.

As I turn the corner, I run into Robb's best friend, Troy. 'Are you still pregnant?' he asks.

'Evidently.'

'Bugger. I had money on today's date.'

'Well, there's still a few hours to go,' I tell him. 'I'll do my best.'

As the days tick by, the messages from friends and family come one after the other: 'Any news?' 'Still preggs?' I walk on the treadmill and watch back-to-back episodes of *Felicity*. Three days past my due date, Robb leaves his phone at home. 'ARE YOU SERIOUS?' I write in the subject line of an email. He replies sheepishly, 'I'll come home at lunch and get it.' He needn't have – still no baby.

Next: the 'helpful' tips. 'SEX. Have you tried sex?' 'Long walks worked for me!' 'There's this special tea …' 'Curries! The hotter the better!'

Each new ache and pain is a sign. *That's interesting*, I think, typing the latest symptom into Google. *Perhaps it's time.*

It isn't time.

The less helpful tips follow. 'Take it from me, you DO NOT want to be induced. My sister's best friend's cousin was induced and they said it hurts SO much more, and you'll end up needing a C-section.' 'Sex! Walk! Tea! Stimulate your nipples!'

The obstetrician pencils in my induction for forty-one weeks plus six days. When I'm five days overdue, my phone-based cheer squad changes tack. 'Enjoy the peace!' 'Go see a movie with Robb!' 'Your life will never be the same after he's here! SLEEP! ENJOY THE FREEDOM.' But I do none of these things.

How to describe this strange absence of emotion? It is as though all my feelings have been stripped of colour. The baby is inside of me, but doesn't really feel part of me, but is somehow also all of me? 'In pregnancy there are two bodies,' writes the psychoanalyst and social psychologist Joan Raphael-Leff, 'one inside the other. Two people live under one skin.' I read that during pregnancy, the heart moves in the body – up and to the side.

I think about the last time I was in a maternity unit – when we visited Bek and Kalen, two-and-a-half years prior. I calculate how old he'd be and wonder where Bek, now classified as a 'care leaver', has ended up, whether she had any more children. For the first time in a long time, I sit in the guilt.

It will get better once the baby is here, I tell myself. I will feel *something* once the baby is here.

I walk and walk and walk and walk and walk.

~

'I was induced with all four of you,' Mum tells me when I call her. I am trying something I saw on a baby forum about inducing labour naturally. It's called curb walking – with one foot on the street, the other in the gutter. 'Evan was a whole two weeks late. Maybe it's genetic.'

On the night before my induction, with no sign of my little womb mate, I order a spicy curry and an orgasm. But curry, sex and three laps around the block in the freezing dark achieves absolutely nothing – not even a lousy Braxton Hicks contraction.

For one last night, I'm kept awake by the morse code of tiny kicks.

~

In the hospital the following morning, the obstetrician breaks my waters with a long silver hook. It's so absurd, so unexpected that, despite my anxiety, I laugh as the hot fluid gushes out, pooling into the towels propped underneath me. With a surfboard-like pad between my legs, we are sent by the obstetrician on a walk around the block to see if it kickstarts my labour. Robb takes my hand as we do laps around the hospital. We stop at the newsagent and I buy a stack of magazines and a packet of jellybeans, armed for the delivery.

The baby kicks and kicks and kicks.

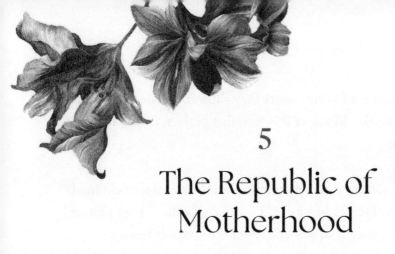

5
The Republic of Motherhood

'Giving birth brings a woman the closest she will ever come to the tender heart of life. Life and death will be right in the room with you, you will feel life's breath upon your face and know the throb of life's blood.'

SUSAN JOHNSON, *A BETTER WOMAN*

We so rarely read about the first few moments after giving birth. There's little written about the space between having a baby and the smiling photos posted to Facebook afterwards, the gushing updates about being 'so in love'. So let me take you there, to that space.

My son is placed on my chest, his beating heart against mine – the miracle of that. He is so much bigger than I thought he would be. It's been months of 'your bump is so small', 'The baby is measuring little', 'He's going to be tiny like his mum'. The weight of him feels all wrong.

Wrenched from between my legs, he is now under my chin. The midwife grabs my breast, places the baby's mouth around it and I lie there, shocked, depleted, a new citizen of what the poet Liz Berry calls 'the Republic of Motherhood'. I wait for the love to come. I wait for the moments they show in movies, the scenes I've read in books. I look at this boy, this perfect, crying boy, and I feel nothing.

Nothing.

Somehow, from somewhere, the platitudes come, ready-made from my lips. 'He's so beautiful,' I say. 'Look at him. He's perfect.' The room is a chorus of yes. I have said the correct lines.

When he doesn't feed, the baby is ripped from me again, passed around the swarm of relatives (when did they arrive?). There's the flash of a camera and the buzz of voices.

As the baby dances around the suite, passed from the crook of one arm to another, the midwife ushers me to the shower. I am bloody, torn, empty. Emptied. I have carried this bump with me for nine months, housed this stranger who knows the rhythm of my heart and the sound of my blood, and now he is gone.

In the shower, the midwife holds me up as I wash the blood from my thighs. I'm high on pethidine, the world spins.

Every birth is different, and I try to make sense of mine, huddled in the shower of that maternity suite, my hair matted, pain emanating from every part of who I am and who I was.

I have wondered in the years since why a post-birth debrief isn't a standard part of delivery, so that someone who was there while you roared your child into the world can fill in the blanks of what happened – or what didn't. Why don't they ask, 'How do you feel? Are you okay? Would you like to talk about your experience?' They could say, 'Yes, your baby is healthy. But for a few minutes his heart rate dropped. That's why the colour drained from the midwife's face and she was commanding you to "PUSH, PUSH!" even though you thought you'd been waiting for the obstetrician.' 'I know that's what we agreed on earlier,' they might say in the moments after, when you're wincing in pain and even blinking hurts, 'that when you started to push we'd call Dr N.' But that's not what happened. No, Dr N was there, shouting, throwing off his watch, donning a blue surgical gown. And you weren't sure why it was happening so fast and why everyone seemed so anxious.

And then it was over. Somehow it was over. The baby was wrenched from your body. And, as the water washes the birth away, you're left in the shower wondering what the fuck just happened.

*

The first night. I wind my hospital bed down until I am lying face to face with my newborn in his clear hospital crib. I think that perhaps if I can see him, if we're on the same level, the love might kick in and I might feel something – anything. I reach out and touch his tiny fingers and toes. Robb has gone home and it's just me and the boy and the pain and a phone alight with messages from family and friends.

We have called him Henry – a family name on both sides and Evan's middle name. Mum said she waited each time until me and my siblings were born before deciding on our names. 'You'll know when you see him,' she said. But I don't know anything.

When I wake to Henry's cries just after midnight, I am drenched. My dressing-gown is soaked through. I wonder, momentarily, if I've wet myself or if the roof is leaking. But it's night sweats. Nobody warned me about night sweats.

It's June – winter solstice, in fact – and I'm freezing. I feed Henry, bones shivering, too sore, too dizzy, *too, too, too,* to get up and change.

In the early hours of the morning a midwife appears, shows me how to change his tiny nappy and swaddles him burrito-tight.

Or did she? Did I dream it?

In the grey light, I heave myself out of bed and limp to the bathroom. 'Cow-heavy', writes Sylvia Plath in her poem 'Morning Song', of early motherhood. Under the fluorescent lighting I lift my top up and stare at my stomach. It is soft, deflated, doughy, the dark *linea nigra* more obvious now my bump has gone. My body hasn't been mine for nine months – but this body isn't mine either. I turn sideways to the mirror and back again, inspecting this new, strange shape. I'm aware of a sharp pain between my legs, of the sweat of the night and the smell of blood.

Why do they only talk about the beauty of motherhood when there is so much horror in it, too?

Years later, I'll see this postpartum body reflected at me for the first time. I am visiting the Art Gallery of NSW for Sydney Dance Company's performance of *Nude Live*. I am part of the nude audience, as naked as the dancers, and writing a piece about it for *The Sydney Morning Herald*. The dancers move in and out of pieces from *Nude: Art from the Tate Collection* while we follow them around from room to room. It's a little bit choose your own adventure – there are solos, pas de deux and group dancers in different spaces, mirroring or responding to the art.

In a moment of stillness I find myself looking at a series of photographs by Dutch photographer Rineke Dijkstra. There are three women, new mothers, captured one hour, one day and one week after giving birth. They are beautiful, vulnerable, shocked. One is pictured with a trickle of blood curling down her inner thigh, while another bears a scar from her C-section.

I stand naked in my own skin, my hand instinctively resting on the belly that sheltered my own son, my boy, and my eyes fill with tears. I am well by then, well enough to work, to dance, to write, but the grief of that time, this time that I am reliving through writing, still takes my breath away.

⁓

The midwives nickname me 'Ms Independent' because I so rarely ask for help. Why can't I ask for help? Why don't I?

'That should have been a red flag,' Dr Q will say, years later.

Mum and Dad visit every day and Robb brings coffee. My younger siblings, Evan, Lulu and Huw, file in after work. They take photos, leave stuffed toys, tiny socks and onesies. My best friend Lizzie comes next, with a bottle of my favourite wine and her glorious rich laugh that I fell in love with when we met during our first week of uni. Her laugh is the sound of my old life, a life before stitches and let-downs, before lochial discharge and after-birth pains. 'He's got the Solomons chin!' Lizzie squeals as Henry sleeps in her arms. She looks up at me, her face aglow. 'He's all you, Arns. He's all you.'

Later, after Lizzie has gone home, I search for the traces of me, the *all me*, in Henry's face. I can't find any.

Unable to sleep, I lie staring at the ceiling. Although I feel a little numb, a little removed, a little not-quite-right, I have not cried. I do not cry. I do not sleep.

'You can get a bit teary when your milk comes in,' Mum says when she visits one evening after work with my beloved Nonna. 'The baby blues. Day three or four is when it usually hits.'

I brace for blue, but all I see is grey.

⁓

'Mother who gave me life,' writes the poet Gwen Harwood. 'I think of women bearing women.' My mother gave me life, but she also gave me a love of literature and poetry, an appreciation for the music of language. She was an English teacher and I spent my childhood rifling through the bookshelves in her study: a collection of HSC texts, such as Peter Goldsworthy's *Maestro* and Marele Day's *The Life and Crimes of Harry Lavender*, crib notes, Shakespeare and stacks of marked student essays. She is beautiful and intelligent and capable. She makes motherhood look easy. She has done this four times. She is a hard act to follow.

Because the baby is so unsettled, one of the midwives brings in a bright pink dummy. I baulk at her suggestion – I am a first-time mother with clear ideas about what I will and will not do, thank you very much (no dummies, no sugar, no TV until age five and even then only educational programming).

'The sucking will help the pressure in his head,' she says, seeing my horrified expression. 'Swelling is pretty common when they use a vacuum during birth.'

A vacuum? Had anyone mentioned a vacuum?

The dummy brings peace. The crying stops. My skull no longer vibrates. It's the first of many 'parenting rules' I break.

In her story 'Giving Birth', Margaret Atwood writes, 'But who gives it? And to whom is it given? Certainly it doesn't feel like giving, which implies a flow, a gentle handing over, no coercion. But there is scant gentleness here.' Nothing about the birth was gentle.

Later, when I go searching for information about instrumental births, I read that the Royal Australian and New Zealand College of Obstetricians and Gynaecologists recommends that new mothers 'be given the opportunity to discuss the reason for operative birth, the management of any complications, and the prognosis for future pregnancies'. Ideally this debrief would happen as soon as possible and be led by the doctor who delivered the baby. (New clinical practice guidelines released in 2023 recommend against 'single-session high-intensity psychological interventions with an explicit focus on re-living the trauma'.)

My memory of these days is blurry, but I don't remember being spoken to about the birth. As soon as the baby arrived, as soon as he was placed in my arms, it was all about him. How many women have heard the line 'All that matters is a healthy baby' while shellshocked from a traumatic birth? How can we expect – or, more importantly, *why* do we expect – new mothers to go through such a life-changing, sometimes life-threatening, experience without stopping to help them understand how they got there?

When I look for the meaning of the word debrief, I am curious about the examples used – a pilot returning from a completed mission, an astronaut returning from space. I think of the poem 'How Becoming a Mother Is Like Space Travel' by Catherine Pierce, one I've shared with other mothers grappling with the enormousness of this transformation.

> *When the astronaut returned*
> *to earth, more tests were run.*
> *Scientists discovered that*
> *seven percent of his genes*
> *had changed in space.*
> *He left the planet*
> *as himself. He came back*
> *as himself, rearranged.*

How to describe this rearrangement of the self that is both instant and ongoing? Matrescence, perhaps, comes closest. I first came across this term in a TED Talk several years ago by the reproductive psychiatrist Dr Alexandra Sacks. But the concept is much older than that. Coined by anthropologist Dana Raphael in her 1975 book *Being Female*, Raphael noted of new motherhood:

> The time of giving birth does not automatically make a mother out of a woman … During this process, this *rite de passage,* changes occur in a woman's physical state, in her status within the group, in her emotional life, in her focus of daily activity, in her own identity and in her relationships with all those around her. The amount of time it takes to become a mother needs study.

In her talk, Sacks built on this remaking: 'When a baby is born so is a mother, each unsteady in their own way. Matrescence is profound but it's also hard and that's what makes it human.'

$\backsim$

I watch the first slippery bath, Robb holding Henry with a gentle strength, guided through the steps by a patient midwife. Midway through, a tour trickles into the room. We become surrounded by expectant parents inspecting the ward.

'Right, so no pressure, then,' Robb jokes and the room fills with laughter. I can tell he is nervous, and I adore him for it. Henry is loved, so loved. For Robb the love has been swift and constant and protective. I can almost see it.

How do you measure love? How do you measure its absence? Like so many mothers (and fathers and partners, too), I expected to feel the rush of love at first sight when I met my baby. More accurately, perhaps, I didn't just expect it – I counted on it.

Why does what we see in movies, on television, in books, differ so wildly from what we know from the research? In an oft-cited study published in 1980 in *The British Journal of Psychology*, 40 per cent of first-time mothers said that their predominant emotion when holding their baby for the first time was indifference. For second-time mothers, it was 25 per cent. Yet there's a prevailing idea that maternal love is biological and instinctual. In a 2018 paper, the authors note that this idea 'clash[es] dramatically' with the reality of what many women experience – and that this leads to feelings of failure, remoteness, shame and guilt.

I become a mother thinking I know all the possible ways that attachment and bonding could go awry – and all the reasons it's so important that it doesn't. So much of child protection work is rooted in attachment theory. The term is thrown around so often – during contact visits, in court documents, in long-term care plans – that it almost loses its meaning, like saying a word over and over again until it's nonsense. 'Indiscriminate attachment', such as the children we removed who were home alone, 'disorganised attachment' (an avoidant attachment style often linked to maltreatment), 'primary attachment' and the catch-all 'attachment difficulties'. In fact, as Sue White and her co-authors argue in their book *Reassessing Attachment Theory in Child Welfare*, the child protection system has 'tended not to be so good at working with all attachment theory's aspects'. 'It has been enthusiastic about using attachment theory to diagnose the deficits,' they note, 'but not so good at recognising love's endurance and prolific reach: love is not a zero-sum game.'

I should be good at this, I think.

ᔥ

'You mean, they're just going to let us leave?' I say to Robb as we get ready for discharge. 'They don't want, like, a note from our mothers or something? A permission slip? Five dollars in a sealed sandwich bag?'

'Looks that way.'

We leave hospital with Henry in his baby capsule. He's dressed in the stripey blue onesie I'd picked out and a white beanie he absolutely hates. It's the first of many sartorial battles to come. I sit in the back next to him as Robb drives us home, slowly, so very slowly.

'Since when do you drive like a little old lady?' I ask.

'Shh,' Robb says. 'I'm concentrating.'

At home, we look at each another and then at the baby. Everything is the same and nothing is the same.

'Right,' says Robb. 'So, what do we do next?'

'Fucked if I know.'

While Henry is sleeping, I go into the bathroom and remove all my clothes. I step onto the scale and look down as the needle adjusts. I weigh almost exactly what I did on my wedding day. I am embarrassed by the relief.

That afternoon, Mum drops over some containers of pasta and salad for dinner. 'The first night at home can be really tough,' she says, shuffling things around in the fridge before sitting down next to me. I hand Henry to her and he sleeps in her arms. He seems happy with her.

In quick succession we're also visited that day by my two aunts, three of my cousins and my sister's new French boyfriend, Pierre, who ignores the baby and takes off on a self-guided tour of our house. My brother Evan and his partner, Amy, come next, stocking our freezer with frozen meals.

I eat the dinner Mum left with one hand while feeding Henry on the couch. My milk has come in and with it a slight fever. I think of Hippocrates, who I once read described postpartum mental illness as 'milk fever' and 'lactation madness'. Mental illness, he said, was a result of breastmilk flowing into the blood. My skin feels hot.

Robb's father flies back from Brisbane to help us finish Henry's room while Robb is on paternity leave. He sleeps on an air mattress downstairs.

Does he notice the tears before I do? They come while I'm changing Henry's nappy. His bottom is covered in tiny red dots.

'The shock of motherhood,' Robb's dad says kindly. 'Jacqui went through exactly the same thing when Bella was born. Why don't you let me hold him for a bit?'

I hand him the baby, who sleeps in his arms. He seems happy with him.

I notice the rash again in the middle of the night while I'm changing the baby's nappy. Is it day six? Day seven?

'You okay, Arns?' Robb calls out.

I switch on the light and inspect the rash closely, conscious of the beat of my heart. Everything is louder when the whole world sleeps.

I touch the red dots – they seem to be multiplying. I smooth on some cream and wonder if it's just the light.

'Arns? Do you need a hand?'

'All good,' I say. 'I'm coming back to bed.'

The next day, a maternal, child and family health nurse from the local early childhood centre knocks on our front door. She introduces herself, and when I let her in I'm aware of how odd it feels, how vulnerable, to allow this stranger into my space to meet my child.

'I'm sorry about the mess,' I tell her, gesturing towards the couch. The living room is full of furniture Robb has stacked together – the change table, which will eventually live in the baby's room, and empty boxes.

'Are you renovating?' Pam says, in a voice that suggests she's seen it all.

'A little, yeah,' I say. 'We'd planned to finish before he came along but ...'

'These things always take longer,' Pam says kindly. 'That nesting urge is strong. What did you say your baby's name was?'

'Henry.'

'Hello, Henry.'

After we've run through whether the baby's sleeping (not much) and feeding (all the time), Pam looks down at my stomach, now flat again, and asks me if I'm remembering to eat. Breastfeeding around the clock has sucked the flesh and muscle from my bones and I am scrawny and gaunt. 'Some mums forget to eat because they're so focused on their babies,' she says. 'But if you're breastfeeding it's very important. Lots of small meals if you can.'

Pam hands me a pen and picks up the baby's Blue Book – the NSW health record given to every new parent.

'Now, what do you do for work?' she asks.

'I'm a psychologist. For DoCS.'

'Oh!' she says, laughing. 'Right. You lot are the worst.'

I laugh, but the comment stings.

While she weighs Henry and writes in his Blue Book, I answer the Edinburgh Postnatal Depression Scale (EPDS).

Or do I? I know now that most women aren't screened until around week four or six because any earlier can give a false positive. Mothers should also be screened on at least one further occasion in the first year of motherhood. So, was I screened early? It's certainly possible.

The EPDS is a standard test designed to screen women for emotional distress during pregnancy and after having a baby. The questionnaire asks them to consider these statements and then rate how they've been feeling in the previous week:

1. I have been able to laugh and see the funny side of things
2. I have looked forward with enjoyment to things
3. I have blamed myself unnecessarily when things went wrong
4. I have been anxious or worried for no good reason
5. I have felt scared or panicky for no very good reason
6. Things have been getting on top of me
7. I have been so unhappy that I have had difficulty sleeping
8. I have felt sad or miserable
9. I have been so unhappy that I have been crying
10. The thought of harming myself has occurred to me

The response scale for some of the questions is oddly poetic.

I have looked forward with enjoyment to things:
a. As much as I ever did
b. Rather less than I used to
c. Definitely less than I used to
d. Hardly at all

The EPDS isn't diagnostic – it doesn't tell you if you're suffering from anxiety or depression. Instead, it's a screening tool for identifying women who may require further care. A score of thirteen (out of a possible thirty) signals the need for a follow-up. And a score of three or less on the last question – which indicates possible suicidal thoughts – requires the clinician to complete a thorough evaluation of the mum's safety.

While it is the most common measure, here and around the world, used to screen for postnatal depression and anxiety, the EPDS is not without its limitations – particularly given that it relies on a mother's own responses. A high score also doesn't mean that a mother will seek treatment.

I can only assume I passed the EPDS with flying colours. Pam says nothing about my score, and I do not ask. I am *fine*, though. Maybe a little anxious, but what new mum isn't? And I, of all people (*you lot*), should know what I'm doing.

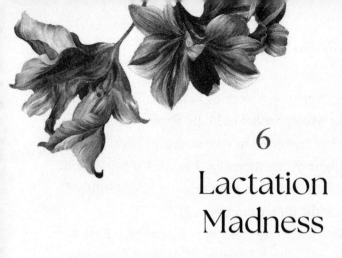

6

Lactation Madness

*'I am glad my case is not serious! But these
nervous troubles are dreadfully depressing.'*
CHARLOTTE PERKINS GILMAN, 'THE YELLOW WALLPAPER'

After just two weeks of parental leave, which feels woefully inadequate (and is, of course), Robb is needed back in the office. As he waves goodbye on that first morning, I feel something I hadn't expected: resentment.

'Your life hasn't changed,' I want to say when I hear the car door close outside and the creak of the old garage door. But I don't. Because I wanted this, wanted this baby, wanted this life (*now, now, now*).

I can't help but feel, though, that Robb's body and mind have remained the same, while mine feel like they belong to someone else. I am simply trying them on for size – and they don't fit quite the way I thought they would.

'It's just you and me, bud,' I tell the baby's head. He doesn't respond. That newborns aren't born conversationalists is just one of many lessons I've already learned.

I check the app I diligently downloaded for sleeping and

feeding (monitoring, tracking, obsessing) and realise I've diligently put him on the wrong boob. I'm Dolly Parton on one side, Kate Moss on the other. Because I'm certain this physical anomaly will be the highlight of my morning, I reach for my phone to text Robb a photo. But my attempt at sending nudes is foiled when I clumsily knock the phone out of reach.

Instead, I complete a delicate transfer mission from Kate to Dolly and switch on morning television. I discover I can now recite the Genie Bra infomercial verbatim. It's a talent, I suspect, that will impress no one.

According to the app, I have about forty-five minutes until the baby requires a refill – enough time to get a coffee. I find the pram collapsed flat by the front door, and panic when I realise I've never actually put it up on my own. We've ventured outside a few times since bringing the baby home, but Robb's always set up the pram.

I twiddle the various levers and buttons. It remains stubbornly closed for business. *You are a competent, educated woman*, I tell myself. *You can do this.* Evidently, though, I can't.

I do what I really didn't want to do: I call Robb at work. He cackles and asks if I'm serious, and then attempts to talk me through it, telling me it's not rocket science, that I've seen him do it before and that the whole reason we bought this pram was because it was so user-friendly. Remember?

'It clearly bloody *is* rocket science because otherwise it wouldn't be so hard,' I tell him.

When I still can't get it working, Robb suggests I google the brand to see if they have a how-to video. They do, of course. A woman with a soothing voice takes me through the steps, making it all sound so easy. And it is. I was simply pressing the wrong button. The pram leaps to attention, ready for service.

Our local café isn't far, but much like Robb on our drive home from hospital, I manoeuvre the pram slowly, carefully, along the footpath.

'He arrived!' Margot, the young café owner, squeals when she spots us. She looks me up and down and raises an eyebrow. 'You don't look like you've had a baby.'

'I *feel* like I've had a baby.'

Margot laughs. 'Fair enough. Double shot today?'

'Yes, please.'

As I pay for my coffee, the baby starts to wail. It's soft at first, a little newborn bleat, but he's been around long enough for me to know where it's going. And it's nowhere good.

'I think he needs a feed, dear.' An elderly woman leans close to the pram, smiling at Henry before fixing her eyes on mine. 'You should feed him.' I feel my face flush with shame. While she wanders off, I calculate whether it would be easier to rush home or whip a boob out on the park bench nearby. The baby's cries get louder, as though he can hear my thoughts.

When we get to the bench, I try to unclip the strap of my feeding singlet. I've yet to attempt breastfeeding outside and the fancy breastfeeding cover Robb's sister Jacqui bought me is back at home. The baby is too small and without the pillows I've been using, I can't seem to hold him properly. He screams louder.

'Okay, bud, let's just get you home,' I say in a low, steady voice, meant for the people walking past. 'I think it's time for a feed.'

Back at home, I cry into a cold muffin while the baby reacquaints himself with Dolly. The crumbs fall into his hair like large pieces of dandruff. The remote control is out of reach (rookie error #1) and I left my phone in my bag (rookie error #2), so I try to follow the plot line of *The Young and the Restless*. Anything to stay awake.

It's not even ten a.m.

৶

Late afternoon, grey light. I am hunched over the change table, wrestling with a nappy, when it occurs to me that night and day no longer matter. Dizzy with exhaustion, drunk with it, I fantasise about sleep. I lust for it. Then panic hits – I have no idea when I *will* sleep again. This baby, this noisy, red-faced stranger, doesn't doze for longer than forty-five-minute stretches.

Thoughts of sleeping are overtaken by thoughts of *not sleeping*, of never sleeping again, and I stand, seized with the terror that nothing makes sense anymore. Time, space, day, night, light, dark – it's all nonsense.

৶

With the baby cocooned in the carrier, I walk around the block and around again. His eyes droop, fighting sleep and seeking sky. My heart may not be working the way it should (*Where is the love? Where is it?*) but he knows the steady music of it, and snuggles close. It is freezing outside but the walls of the house are closing in on me. Who knew babies' cries could take up so much space?

In the fierce wind I think of the poet Robert Frost's lines:

> *And miles to go before I sleep,*
> *And miles to go before I sleep.*

Before I sleep before I sleep before I sleep sleep sleep sleep sleep sleep
As I round the block again, half conscious on shaky legs, my phone vibrates. A text from a newly engaged friend: 'How are you??? Is it the most wonderful thing you've ever experienced?!' Her words make me violently angry. I am the first of my friends

to have a baby and I'm furious to be carrying the burden of this secret life alone.

I write back after four days, 'Yes! I'm exhausted, but yes!'

I don't hear from her again for months. The silence is a slap. Later, I'll find out she was offended it took me so long to reply.

⌇

At 3.45 a.m. I google: *Can you die from lack of sleep?*

I am certain there is something wrong with the baby, something I don't know how to articulate. I can't make out his features. I look at his nose and the rest of his face is out of focus. There is no 'whole', only parts. I could be looking after someone else's child. Sometimes I wonder if I am.

Sometimes I wonder when his mother is coming to get him.

⌇

When Robb gets home from work, he sits up with the baby so I can shower and clutch at something that resembles sleep. I try to rest from eight p.m. until midnight, enough to make it through the sleepless hours until dawn. Only it's not enough; it's not even close. I lie awake, my breasts tingling with the strange sensation of producing milk.

The baby won't sleep unless he's being held, so we take turns cradling him. I'm too scared I will suffocate him accidentally if I bring him into our bed, having been indoctrinated in the child protection mantra of 'no co-sleeping'. And so, we learn to divide and conquer.

But while it makes logistical sense, I miss my husband madly. Fatigue makes us shorter with one another, playfulness pushed aside for practicality. Survival. We pass in the hallway like zombies and argue over the littlest things. I miss the 'us' we were. Why did I think we needed more? This is not more. I have ruined everything.

ℭ

The baby is three weeks old. After weeks of one smooth feed after another, everything changes. He arches and cries in my lap, latching on and off and on. I switch him around and try the other side. He cries. I cry.

On one of his afternoon visits, while we drink tea and watch the news, Dad suggests trying to feed the baby on an angle. 'Here,' he says, grabbing some cushions from the couch and demonstrating. 'Like this.'

I try. It fails. The baby and I cry together.

ℭ

In the folder of paperwork from the hospital, I learn that our Early Childhood Centre has a breastfeeding clinic at eleven a.m. on Wednesday mornings. I bundle the baby into the pram and walk the twenty minutes to the centre. I haven't driven since he was born, too tired to get behind the wheel. The sky is too blue, too bright.

Inside one of the rooms, there are six other new mothers in various stages of undress. It feels a bit like a live breastfeeding masterclass, boobs out, nurses walking around correcting our technique like ballet masters. ('Sit up straight. Tummy in. Once again, but I want you to really *feel* it this time.') I find an empty chair and set myself up.

'How old is yours?' the woman beside me asks.

'Three weeks,' I say. 'I think?'

She laughs. 'I know what you mean.'

Do you, though? I wonder. She looks happy, together, like she's managed to shower and get dressed more than once in the last week. The baby, who has not fed properly for days, latches on perfectly.

'He's not usually like this,' I tell one of the nurses. 'See, normally he thrashes around and latches on and off, and he cries. He cries a lot. It's not usually like this.'

'Sometimes it's because there are other babies around,' the nurse says. 'What a cutie. Keep it up, mum.'

'But there aren't any other babies at home,' I want to say. 'It's just me and the walls, and the crying and the crying and my useless boobs and for god's sake help me.' But I don't. I just pack up my pram and leave.

Back at home, with Wendy Kingston reading the afternoon news bulletin as my witness, it all goes to shit. I scour FAQs and troubleshooting tips via Dr Google, as if my breasts are a malfunctioning white good.

'He just won't latch on,' I text my mum. 'Did you ever have this problem?'

'Oh no, I never had any problems,' she texts back between students. 'Are you still having trouble? Gosh, I remember breastfeeding one of you while cooking dinner. Probably Huw?? I'll call you later xx.'

Despite my experience with helplines, I have never phoned one myself. But I am desperate. Nothing seems to be working.

The woman on the Australian Breastfeeding Association helpline diagnoses me with an oversupply issue. 'I think your milk is coming out too fast. Have you tried lying down?'

Have I tried lying down? I have tried everything.

I find the phone number for Janet, a lactation consultant, on a list provided by the early childhood nurse. She says she'll come to the house and asks me to keep some of the baby's nappies. When Janet arrives, she inspects the nappies with gloved hands, frowns, and passes judgement on the quality of my milk.

'You have a foremilk/hindmilk issue,' she says.

'A what?' Breastfeeding is a language I do not understand. It has arrived in my life 'like hieroglyphs from the land of the lost', as Maggie Nelson writes in *The Argonauts*. Breastfeeding is a dance with steps I cannot pick up. And I've always been able to dance.

'It means he's not getting enough of the good stuff that comes later in the feed. The fatty milk.'

'Oh. Right.'

'And you need to stop drinking coffee and eating tomatoes.'

'Why can't I eat tomatoes?'

'Too acidic, love.'

When I tell the paediatrician about our feeding problems at the six-week check-up, he tells me the baby has reflux and pre-scribes Mylanta and Losec.

'Mylanta?' I ask. 'You mean like normal Mylanta, Mylanta?'

'Exactly. And how are YOU, mum?' he asks. I bristle at 'mum'. I have a name, too.

'Tired.'

The paediatrician nods – it's the correct answer. All new mums are tired.

I want to tell him that there is something else wrong with the baby. I don't know how to explain it, though, don't know how to explain what is so clear yet so unclear at the same time. So I don't try. I don't try.

At home, I shoot the bright blue liquid into the baby's mouth with a syringe.

The crying doesn't stop. He doesn't put on any weight.

Awake. Pacing, patting, bouncing, singing, begging.

Asleep. Wired, wired, wired, wired.

I check my phone; it's after two a.m. I learn that Amy Winehouse has died.

Google, three a.m.: *How do I put my baby up for adoption?*

The DoCS website is the first result. I close the tab.

〜

'I hope you're not cleaning for me,' says my friend Brooke, peering through the screen door on her first visit to meet the baby. I've known Brooke since primary school and she's one of my oldest friends. She's no-nonsense, practical and loyal, and has just returned from a stint living overseas.

'God no,' I tell her. 'I mean, I love you, but not enough to clean. The vacuum's the only thing that will get him to sleep.'

Brooke laughs before handing me a blue gift bag and a tray with two coffees.

'You'd think the house would be spotless by now,' I say, 'but there's an app that just plays vacuum sounds on loop, so I don't actually have to do anything.'

'Whatever works, right?'

'Exactly.'

'So, how's motherhood?' Brooke asks, sitting next to me on the couch while I breastfeed. 'Do you love it?' Robb's cat hisses at her and runs away. She smirks. 'And how's the evil cat going with the baby?'

'She seems to know her place,' I say. 'Weirdly.'

'And you?' Brooke says again. 'What's wrong with your eye?'

'Oh, it's nothing,' I reply. But it's not nothing – I had noticed it earlier, a burst blood vessel blooming in the corner of my left eye. 'I mean, we're not getting any sleep, so it's probably from that. But we're so lucky, you know? He's perfect.' I burp the baby and hand him over to her.

'He's pretty cute.' Brooke smiles and pulls his singlet down over his tummy while I head to the kitchen for a glass of water. The baby is rarely settled for long, and these moments of silence are scarce. 'Oh my god,' Brooke says suddenly. 'Did I tell you Annabel and Rick broke up?'

Later that evening, the vacuum app buzzes as Robb and I are shovelling down some dinner before the baby starts crying again.

'Will he be twenty-two years old and still soothing himself to sleep with a vacuum noise app?' I say to Robb. 'Maybe? Do we care?'

'No, we do not.'

✑

After weeks of one-sided conversation, the first gummy smile is a gift – a tiny, luminous gift. Robb is greedy for them, too, and when I watch him with the baby, the weight of my heart lifts, ever so slightly. I can still feel love for Robb. I am capable of it. I have never loved my husband more. And yet there's a baby-shaped piece of love missing. *What the fuck is wrong with me?*

When the baby is eight weeks old, Robb flies to Los Angeles for ten days. He's leading a business unit at Disney, and now that the baby is here he's expected to travel again. It's his first trip away since my pregnancy and comes far too soon. I send Robb photographs of the baby in his bouncer and post them to Facebook.

'Man of the house while Daddy's away.' (Sixteen likes / eight comments / no shares.)

I don't have a mother's group yet and my friends and family

are all at work. I have never felt so lonely – I am also never alone.

How did I keep us both alive? I find these words on the notes app in my phone, written three years ago when I began trying to piece together what happened and when. How did I keep us both alive?

Existing somewhere between awake and asleep, I bring the baby to bed with me, pushing the mattress up against the wall so he can't fall off. When I do sleep, I wake swatting the sheets, terrified I've rolled onto him in the night.

This is such a common occurrence that researchers have given it a name: the baby-in-bed nightmare pattern. A mother searches through the covers, cries, calls out. She grabs her partner, yells at him to look. And when awake, and having realised the baby isn't with her, she'll often still rise to check on them. 'Such behaviours may reflect a mother's state of maternal vigilance; they may even serve a functional role in her infant caregiving,' reports one study.

But I don't know this then, waking in the night, sweat-soaked and frightened.

Because Robb knows I won't, he puts a call out on Facebook asking people to please drop in and see me and the baby while he's overseas. It annoys me; I bat most of the requests away except from my cousin Bryn, with whom I've always been close. He visits with his boyfriend and a lasagne.

'You weren't yourself,' Bryn says when I asked him recently about the visit. 'There was a faraway look in your eyes. That's what I remember.'

⟳

'It's bad, isn't it? It's really bad.' I snap a photo of the rash on Henry's bottom and send it to Robb in LA. It has multiplied again – red spots of varying sizes. Every time I look at it, it seems worse. I don't know what time it is over there, but Robb doesn't respond straight away. Still, I send another, then another, all different angles of the same angry rash.

My hands shake. Sweat pools in my armpits. I have tried nappy-free time (like the websites say). I have squirted breast-milk onto the rash (like the websites say). I have covered him with the thick white cream we got in the baby bags from hospital (like the websites say).

But nothing is working. Every time the doorbell rings, I think the social workers are here to take him and I lie on the kitchen floor until they leave. I pull the curtains shut. I switch off all the lights.

Always sight the child.

They're coming for him. The nappy rash is so bad, they're going to come and remove him, and everyone will know what a terrible, terrible failure of a mother you are.

'Did you ask your dad?' Robb finally texts later. 'I'm sorry, I've been so flat out. I love you. It looks okay to me. Are you using the Sudocrem? Did Brooke come by?'

They're coming for him. I know it. I deserve it. It's my turn.

᠅

The baby is eleven weeks old when our first mothers' group meets at the Early Childhood Centre in Waterloo. I had just missed the cut-off for the earlier group, so it's later than usual. I don't particularly want to go. I've heard nothing but terrible stories about competitive, mean-girl mothers, but I force myself to get dressed and leave the house.

As I get closer to the centre, I realise it's near to where three years ago Jo and I had dropped off two scared girls with very little English to their grandmother after we had removed them from their dad. I remember a belt, a laceration to the face, a father in the office downstairs who, highly intelligent, sparred with me over the semantics of our allegations. I remember losing my temper, nerves frayed, uncharacteristically hitting the desk.

I didn't like the way it was changing me.

I consider turning back – there are parts of the city, parts where we used to do home visits, that make me feel ill. But I am almost there. And I am lonely.

The babies in the group are all boys except for little Bea, who has bright blue eyes and, according to her (apologetic) mum, Angela, has slept through the night since she was six weeks old. We introduce ourselves and share birth stories. There are tears, but there's laughter, too.

At the end of the hour, when the nurses ask us if we have any questions, Angela says, 'Just wondering, if I'm breastfeeding, when can I have a glass of wine?'

Everyone laughs. The ice is broken.

'You have a supply issue,' says a GP I've never seen before, when I tell her the Mylanta doesn't seem to be working and I'm not sure when I last slept for more than forty-five minutes.

She prescribes Motilium, a medication used 'off-label' to increase lactation. It works almost immediately. Within forty-eight hours, my milk is abundant; my breasts ache. I stuff cold cabbage leaves down my bra to soothe the pain. But although my breasts leak and hurt to touch, the baby still thrashes and cries. My mouth breaks out in cold sores.

I stop taking the Motilium pills. My milk supply dwindles.

I don't have enough to feed him.

He wakes hourly overnight.

He loses more weight.

His skin looks grey.

Mum would sing to us when she put us to bed, so I try singing to the baby. I remember her voice in the dark – falling asleep to 'Scarborough Fair'. But my song is a plea: please stop crying. Please.

Sleep while the baby sleeps, they say; sleep while the baby sleeps. But what if the baby never sleeps? What if the baby never fucking sleeps?

When I look at the baby, I see a collision of features that don't make any sense. He appears foreign and far away – a face of shapes I can't decipher. Sometimes, he turns into a dragon. The first time was a shock – a little green dragon lying on the play mat doing tummy time. But it's more frequent now: a little green dragon in a highchair; a little green dragon in the pram. Just a flash and then it's gone.

I take photo after photo trying to capture what I see. And what I don't.

'You used to call him "dragon baby",' Robb will say, years later. 'I didn't realise you meant it literally.'

It's Saturday and Robb has gone to the office for a few hours. I take the baby for a walk through the back streets of Darlington, our usual quiet route. Today, though, the markets are on at Carriageworks and I'm overwhelmed by the number of people on the pavement. I never used to be worried about crowds, but now all the voices and oversized bunches of flowers are too loud, too loud, too loud. I put my head down and push through with the pram.

'Ariane!' I look up. It's Delia, one of the mums from my mothers' group. Her baby is strapped to her chest. We haven't met up many times, but we've texted a little.

'Hi,' I say, grateful for a familiar face. 'How are you going?'

'I'm good,' she says. 'Finally getting a bit more sleep, which helps.' Delia gestures to the man next to her. 'Ariane, this is my husband, Mark. Mark, this is Ariane.' She smiles and points towards Henry. 'And that's Henry. Isn't he adorable? Look at those cheeks and blue eyes.'

I look down at what Delia's looking at and back up at her. She's still smiling.

But he isn't really adorable. And I can't understand why no one will tell me the truth.

∽

In the third mothers' group meeting, right in the middle of a talk about sleep and settling, the baby starts to cry.

'I'm sorry. He's not exactly a fan of either,' I joke, attempting to shove a nipple into his mouth. He rejects it, rejects me. I try the other side. He rejects it, rejects me. When I can't calm him, I leave the room like a naughty school student. It's exactly what happens when we feed at home, but in public I am humiliated.

One of the early childhood nurses follows me. I burst into tears while she takes the baby from my arms and sways, bounces, pats.

'Do you mind if I watch you feed?' she asks. I nod, sitting on one of the chairs. I'm crying so hard I can hardly see. This time, unlike in the breastfeeding masterclass, the baby arches his back, screams, bats at me. We both cry louder.

'Hon, he's got a tongue-tie,' the nurse says finally. She sounds pleased with herself, as though she's successfully cracked another cold breastfeeding case. 'He can't latch on properly. That's why he's having trouble feeding.'

'But the paediatrician said it wouldn't affect feeding,' I say. 'That's what he told me when he was born. God, I'm so tired. I've tried everything.'

'You can't feed him with that tongue-tie, hon. Come on, come and have a seat in my office.'

The nurse makes me a cup of tea and offers me a biscuit. I am high on the endorphins of too many tears.

'I can give you the name of the tongue-tie clinic,' she says. 'But there might be a bit of a wait. Or you can try pumping and bottle-feeding. It can be time-consuming, though. A lot of work and a lot of cleaning. And I can see you're already exhausted.' She smiles at the baby. 'You can also use formula, of course. I think you should be topping up with some formula.'

As the other mothers file out, Angela shoots me a smile and gestures that she'll call.

None of the other mums are using formula, I think as I watch them leave with their prams. *Literally none. What is so wrong with you?*

When Robb gets home from work later that day, I tell him, 'He was starving!' I am sitting on the couch, yelling over the whirr of the yellow breast pump. 'That's why he won't stop crying. I was fucking starving him.'

But I am not ready to give up, not ready to formula-feed, not completely. This is absurd to me now, looking back. What was I trying to prove?

I pump around the clock, just like the early childhood nurse told me in the notes she scribbled onto a piece of paper. When I am not bottle-feeding, I am pumping. I am pumping for Australia.

My supply, however, is pitiful, and when I accidentally spill a hard-won 50-millilitre bottle all over the kitchen bench, it sends me into a rage.

'No use crying over spilt milk,' Robb says, trying to make me laugh.

'Too soon,' I snap. 'Too fucking soon.'

It hadn't occurred to me that I would do anything other than excel at breastfeeding. The thought hadn't even crossed my Type A mind. How could I possibly fail at something so 'natural'? I went to the breastfeeding seminar at the maternity hospital, I read the relevant chapter in *What to Expect*. I even studied the various positions on the breastfeeding pamphlet as though they were choreography I could mimic – cradle hold, cross-cradle hold, football hold. But nothing is working.

'Parenthood isn't a test you can ace,' an anaesthetist friend later tells me. Breastfeeding isn't either. And while we might have moved passed the idea of 'milk fever', we know from research that women who struggle with breastfeeding may be at increased risk for postnatal depression. But research also shows that intentions matter, too – one study found that women who *wanted* to breastfeed but couldn't had higher rates of depression. Not everyone wants to breastfeed, of course, but the pressure to do so is immense. The World Health Organization recommends breastfeeding until the baby is two years old; we're told that breastfeeding is 'free' (if you ignore the economic, time and psychological costs of pumping and seeing lactation consultants); and more recently the message is that by using fewer resources and producing minimal waste, breastfeeding is better for the planet.

Not being able to breastfeed 'properly' only adds to the ways I feel I'm already failing as a mother. When I buy formula, I bury it in the bottom of the pram under the nappy bag, where no one can see my secret shame.

∽

'You should take a photo of yourself feeding,' says Megan, my former child protection boss, when I text her that I'm weaning and feeling both sadness and relief. She's one of the few people I know who has a baby around the same age. 'It might seem strange,' she texts, 'but you might like to look back on it.' And so I do – a blurry selfie of Henry feeding in the dark on the couch.

When I find the photo years later, all I can see is how dead my eyes were, how vacant I looked. Megan was right, though – I'm glad I have it. We really did try our best.

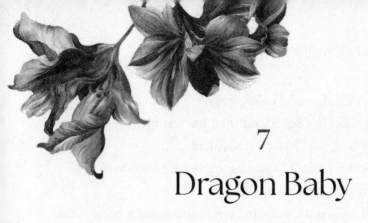

7

Dragon Baby

'It's true what they say, that a baby gives you a reason to live. But, also, a baby is a reason that it is not permissible to die. There are days when this does not feel good.'

RIVKA GALCHEN, *LITTLE LABOURS*

In the fridge section of the supermarket in Waterloo, I am trying to work out what I've come to the shops for. We're out of food – I know that much. I told Robb I'd pick up ingredients to make dinner, but I can't remember a single recipe. I lift the light-green muslin wrap off the pram so the baby can extend his legs. He's been a dragon for most of the morning – a quiet, happy dragon, though, engrossed in the discovery of his right big toe. I notice the arches of his feet with a detached sense of pride – they're high like a dancer's, high like mine.

We've been alone until now, in the quiet hours of a midweek morning. But I'm aware of a young couple, a girl and a boy, walking towards us, their swinging hands clasped together. The girl is in her early twenties and looks down at the baby then up at her boyfriend. She points at him, whispers something, laughs.

'What are you looking at?' I snap, staring at her.

The girl frowns and looks at the baby. 'Sorry?'

'What do you think you're looking at?'

The girl glances at her boyfriend then back at me.

'Sorry,' she says, again. 'I just – he looked cold.'

'Are you a mum?' I ask. 'Do you have any idea how hard it is?'

'Sorry. I really didn't mean anything.'

I watch the couple walk away, the boyfriend peering back over his shoulder.

Hands shaking, I call Robb from the canned food aisle.

'Arns?' he says. 'You okay?'

'I'm in the supermarket,' I whisper. 'They were looking at him, this couple. And I just lost it. Shit. I'm so embarrassed. I yelled at her. My hands are still shaking. I have to get out of here. I don't think I can buy dinner. I don't want to run into them again.'

'Don't worry, I'll get something on the way home,' Robb says. 'Why don't you head back to the house and I'll come home early?'

'Okay.'

Head down, I put my empty basket back at the front of the store.

'I'm sorry,' I say to Robb over the noise of the traffic. 'I tried.'

'I know you did,' Robb says. 'I love you.'

⁊

'Henry is so cute, Arns,' Brooke tells me one evening, when she drops by after work. I have stopped letting people come over – I must protect the baby from prying eyes – but I have made an exception for Brooke.

Robb is overseas again. She pushes the pram for me while we walk around the streets of Redfern, lined with scruffy terraces and large council bins. Brooke's friend has just had a baby and she tells me how 'funny looking' he is.

'It's weird,' she says. 'And this is mean, I know. Both parents are attractive, too. But he looks like a grumpy old man. Henry is super cute, though.'

I look down into the pram, into the mess of features in front of me, and back at her. The baby's not a dragon today, but he still doesn't look right somehow.

'It's okay,' I snap at Brooke. 'You don't have to lie to me.' I take the pram from her, trying not to show how angry I am. 'I know he's not cute,' I say. 'You of all people don't have to pretend.'

I am so tired of having to pretend when everyone around me is lying. Why am I the only one trying to protect him?

Brooke laughs, then stops and stares at me.

'Wait, you're being serious?' she says. She looks down at the baby, then back up at me. We keep walking towards the house.

'Arns,' she says, her voice lower than usual, 'do you think it's weird you don't think your own baby is cute?'

'I don't know,' I tell her. My voice is a challenge. What would she know? 'Is it?'

Later, after she's gone home, Brooke texts me the number for the PANDA helpline and a link to their website.

'Thanks!' I reply. 'I'll take a look!'

I don't.

⁓

In her incredible novel *Nightbitch,* a book I've returned to again and again, Rachel Yoder describes the intense isolation of new motherhood. The loneliness of her main character, whom we know as Nightbitch, feels almost tangible, 'as if it were her second child'. In one scene Nightbitch describes a group of mothers with their bagged snacks, sniffing nappies and running after children with tissues. There's a look, she continues, that all mothers have – a combination of boredom, exhaustion and grief for what and who they've lost. Nightbitch actively avoids making mum friends because although she's a mum, she's not *that kind* of mum.

Most local mothers' groups bring vulnerable women together based on their postcode and their child's date of birth. But while nothing bonds women faster than sharing birth stories (while still bleeding and leaking and reeling), there's often an element of performance when meeting new people – and particularly so as a new mother. There's a level of loneliness about this that I couldn't quite articulate until years later.

'This is not who I am,' I wanted to tell the other mums when I managed to drag myself to Redfern Park, where we'd sit on rugs under the shadows of the trees. 'You didn't know me before and this version of me isn't really me but it's the only me left over. I am not myself, you see.'

$\backsim$

A week before Christmas, Robb and I go to Brooke's birthday party. I blow-dry my hair and wear a long, tight black dress. It's the first time I've been out at night since the baby was born six months ago. Underweight and out of practice, I drink too much too quickly.

Another couple have brought their baby, a boy born ten days before Henry. He is longer and thinner than Henry and has a mop of blond curls. When he's passed to me, I hand him quickly to Robb. 'I don't want to hold him,' I whisper. 'I've already got one at home.' Robb hands the baby to the woman next to me, squeezes my hand.

After dinner I stand with two younger couples, both newly married. They ask polite questions about motherhood and maternity leave – how I'm finding it, how long I'm taking off work.

'Yeah, it's pretty hard,' I say. 'I mean, if I knew then what I know now, I'm not sure I would have done it.' There's an awkward silence and I laugh too loudly. 'I mean, totally worth it, obviously! It's great. Love him!'

Later, in the car, my eyes are scratchy with fatigue and my head is full of wine. 'I reckon you might have been a bit too honest,' Robb says. 'Like, I reckon you've put them all off having babies.'

'Well, no one told me any of this,' I say, sulking. 'Someone has to tell the truth.'

Google, 3.57 a.m.: *Does motherhood get any easier?*

⌁

It occurs to me as I'm out walking one afternoon, pushing the pram around and around and around, that I don't actually exist. I am dead. I have already died. If I don't actually exist, then it won't matter if I kill myself, because you can't kill something that never existed. And if I am already dead, then no one will miss me. It feels as though I have solved some great puzzle of life and death – all the pieces of existence have fallen into place. I am calm. I am so very calm.

Around and around and around and around and around and around and around.

Years later, trying to understand how I could feel both alive and dead, I read a report about a woman who experienced Cotard's delusion ten days after her baby was born. The condition is characterised by nihilistic delusions commonly around the loss of body organs or believing one has died.

'My organs do not work,' she said. 'They rotted, there is nothing inside.'

I am hollow.

∾

'I can't get up,' I tell Robb one morning from bed. 'I … I just can't seem to get up.' My limbs feel like concrete. Tears leak out of the corner of my eyes. I can't lift my head. It is too heavy for me.

'It's okay,' Robb says, taking the baby from my leaden arms. 'You need to sleep. Get some sleep. I'll go in late or work from home.'

And he's right. He's always right. I'm just tired. I just need sleep. When did I last sleep? I don't sleep anymore. I don't sleep.

∾

It is 1959. Radio DJ Peter Tripp has been awake for seventy-two hours, three days into his goal of 201 hours. Tripp is raising money for charity, stationed in a clear booth in Times Square. The hallucinations are becoming more vivid: scurrying mice and kittens, a desk drawer on fire, his shoes full of cobwebs. Soon, Tripp is convinced he is an imposter. After 201 hours, he sleeps.

In 1963, teenager Randy Gardner stays awake even longer – 264 hours, or eleven days – as part of a school science experiment. His attempt is more scientifically robust than Tripp's: he does it drug-free and, eventually, under the supervision of sleep researcher William Dement. He becomes moody, hallucinates, loses short-term memory.

Guinness World Records no longer accepts entries for the longest periods spent without sleeping, due to its health impacts.

∽

'In case you need some comic relief,' my brother Evan's partner, Amy, texts me as I'm writing this chapter, 'do you remember when you were so tired you tried to puree raw carrot and broke the baby food machine?'

'No recollection at all,' I text back. 'But that tracks.'

∽

Robb and I have a fight – who knows what it was about now. I throw a plate to the ground as I'm emptying the dishwasher and it shatters over the kitchen tiles.

Robb puts the baby in the pram, straps him in and slams the door. The house shakes.

I am alone in a space that is at once too small and too large.

I need to see the sea. I need to see the sea.

The urge comes from nowhere and then I am, almost trance-like, on a train to Circular Quay.

I need to see the sea.

Down at the harbour, though, there are tourists and families and horns and seagulls and buskers and seagulls and horns and tourists and families and I am back on the train and back at home and back in bed where Robb will find me and kiss me awake.

'I needed to see the sea,' I tell him. 'I don't know why. I needed to see the sea. I'm sorry.'

'I'm sorry, too.'

∽

'If the womb is too moist, the brain is filled with water, and the moisture running over the eyes, compels them to involuntarily shed tears,' wrote thirteenth-century physician Trotula of Salerno in one of the earliest descriptions of postnatal depression.

My brain is full of water.

⟋

In January, Robb flies back to LA for a week. I start crying the moment he leaves for the airport – and I don't stop for three days. Up until then, I have not cried so much as felt numb and empty. I have prided myself on my ability to keep it together for the baby, but now, as I sob over the change table, I know I need help. I can't seem to switch off the tears. They fall off my face, two by two like marching ants.

I tell Robb I'll go and see a doctor and that I'll text Lizzie. She's just returned home from living in Berlin with her husband.

'Your friends want to help, Arns,' Robb says. 'Please let them help while I'm away. They're all really worried about you. Brooke says you haven't texted her back at all. She's messaged me a few times saying she's worried about you.'

'She did?' This angers me. I feel spied on. 'What did she say?'

'That you didn't seem yourself the last time she saw you and that you haven't contacted her since.'

Lizzie comes over to hold the baby while I call to make an appointment with my GP.

'Oh, my love,' she says to me, bouncing him on her hip. 'I'm so glad you called.' Lizzie gets me a blanket and drapes it over me. While she feeds the baby a bottle, I fall into a half-sleep. Half conscious, I hear her speaking and singing to him, the sound of her voice a balm.

When I wake up, Lizzie says, 'Pick a feeling.' It's a phrase we learnt from one of my favourite ballet films, *The Turning Point* with Shirley MacLaine and Anne Bancroft. We've used it through heartbreak and love and grief and illness in the ten years we've been friends.

'Sad,' I say. 'I am just so sad.'

The baby is seven months old, and I am getting worse. My weight has dropped to 45 kilograms, my limbs feel like lead and I am so, so slow. I can't read. I can't find the right words. They stumble off my tongue and disappear.

I didn't know that depression could physically hurt. I knew it was a mental illness, that it lives somewhere in the brain. While working at DoCS I'd seen parents with severe mental illness, visiting them in acute mental health units where they were so unwell they could sometimes barely speak. And yet I had no idea just how physical it could be. On bad days, my left side aches, somewhere in the pit of me. Cover my stomach with sticky gel and you'll see it there on an ultrasound. It aches. Pulses. A dull, localised pain. I want it surgically removed.

On other days it's in my throat. It hurts to swallow. Everything is too noisy, too fast, too violent. I can't keep up. I misjudge the speed of oncoming traffic when I'm crossing the road. I'm too slow as I walk through the barrier at the train station. It slams in front of me before I can pass. There's a thump of metal. I am locked out.

I don't understand my reflection. There are bones in her shoulders that I don't recognise.

Did I eat today? Yesterday? I've lost my hunger. I don't know where I left it.

My eye sockets throb.

I do not want to be alive anymore.

〜

'Don't Trust Your Tired Self,' flashes the sign above a busy inter-section. It's a NSW government campaign warning of the dangers of driving while fatigued. 'Being awake for 17 hours or more has a similar effect on your driving as a blood alcohol con-tent of 0.05.'

And yet, I think, *we ask mothers to mother – to keep another little person alive.*

Don't Trust Your Tired Self.
Don't Trust Your Self.
    You're Tired.

〜

'I still remember taking baby Hen out for a walk,' Amy tells me, 'and when we came back you were in a kind of slow-motion panic that you'd lost him again.'

I am hunting memories, other people's recollections, hoping they might nudge some of my own.

'I had forgotten he was with you?'

'Yeah. I don't think you'd even remembered I had come over. You looked confused when I came to the door with the pram. But then even when you looked in the pram, right at him, you didn't seem to see, you just kept looking for him. I panicked that I had somehow let him fall out of the pram. I didn't know what the fuck was going on. It was surreal. I rationalised it as just total exhaustion. I now feel so awful about how frightened and lonely you must have felt. I'm ashamed I didn't grasp the gravity of the situation.'

'No one did,' I say.

'I know. But it's hard remembering without wanting to slap former me across the face. I mean, seriously? Couldn't see the physical baby?! In what world could tiredness explain that?'

'I don't remember that at all,' I say. 'Not at all.'

∽

Dr Wilson, whom I've seen a few times with the baby, prescribes Zoloft, an SSRI, while I howl into a wad of tissues. He has light green eyes and tells me he has four children, including a daughter the same age as Henry. It's the first time I'm seeing him as a patient myself.

'I don't need you to fill out a form to see you're depressed,' Dr Wilson says softly. So I don't fill out a form. I sit, stunned. He pulls a box of toys down from the bookshelf for the baby and hands me another tissue. He's right – I tell him I can't sleep, can't eat, can't concentrate. I feel numb. Helpless. Lost. Tick, tick, tick, tick. It's a textbook case of severe postnatal depression.

'Are you still breastfeeding?' he asks.

'No. I failed at that. Gave it up. Gave up pumping, too. Couldn't get enough.'

'You didn't fail, Ariane,' he says. 'Breastfeeding is very hard.'

I shrug.

'Are you having any thoughts of harming yourself or Henry?' Dr Wilson asks. His voice is so kind it makes me ache.

'No,' I lie. 'Nothing like that.'

'Alright, then. We're going to get you better.'

∽

In my second-last year of uni, I remember Tom Cruise publicly criticising Brooke Shields for taking medication for her postnatal depression. It came up during an abnormal psychology tutorial, around the time we were learning about psychiatric drugs. In her memoir, *Down Came the Rain*, Shields had shared her experience of postnatal depression after the birth of her first baby, Rowan.

'These drugs are dangerous,' Cruise said in an interview with Matt Lauer on NBC's *Today*. 'I have actually helped people come off. When you talk about postpartum ... there is a hormonal thing that is going on, scientifically, you can prove that. But when you talk about emotional, chemical imbalances in people, there is no science behind that. You can use vitamins to help a woman through those things.'

In an op-ed for *The New York Times*, Shields fired back: 'I'm going to take a wild guess and say that Mr. Cruise has never suffered from postpartum depression. I wasn't thrilled to be taking drugs. In fact, I prematurely stopped taking them and had a relapse that almost led me to drive my car into a wall with Rowan in the backseat. But the drugs, along with weekly therapy sessions, are what saved me – and my family.'

I think of this exchange when I read through the list of side effects on the leaflet with my SSRI: agitation, nervousness, anxiety, frightening dreams, yawning, abnormal thinking, teeth grinding, symptoms of agitation, dizziness, headache, nausea ...

I think about what it means that I need to be medicated in order to mother.

It's another three days before I take the first tablet.

❧

'Your dad said you seemed really flat today,' Mum says on the phone one afternoon. Robb is still away and she and my sister are coming over to visit. Dad's already been and gone, holding Henry while I showered. 'And thin,' she adds. 'He's worried you look thin.'

'I'm depressed, Mum,' I snap. 'I'm fucking depressed. I haven't slept since he was born. I can't feed my own baby. He rejects me. I'm taking antidepressants, for fuck's sake. Thank you for finally noticing that I haven't been myself.'

I am crying and she is crying and the baby is crying and she is saying I didn't know, why didn't you say anything? Why didn't you ask for help? Why didn't you tell me? And she is driving over to my house with dinner and a box of cupcakes, really beautiful, fancy, expensive cupcakes and they are ridiculous because what are we celebrating? But – because when did I last eat properly? – I eat them all and we are sitting on the couch and she is holding the baby and we are both wincing from our failures.

∽

The year I was born, in Camperdown in 1983, was the same year a group of volunteers with lived experience of postnatal depression set up the PANDA helpline. It was also the same year the first mother and baby psychiatric unit opened in Australia, in Larundel, Victoria.

'Postpartum depression kind of didn't really exist,' Professor Anne Buist, an Australian perinatal psychiatrist, tells me when I ask her about what it was like to mother while depressed at this time. 'People didn't know what it was.' And, she tells me, not only did people not know what postnatal depression was, there were no SSRIs to treat it.

'We didn't talk about it,' Mum says when I ask her. 'And I didn't experience anything like it either. But it just wasn't something anyone talked about.'

∽

Along with prescribing an SSRI, Dr Wilson refers me to a perinatal psychiatrist. I leave Henry with Robb and catch the bus into the city. I arrive early, far too early, and walk through the park in the sunshine. When I catch the lift upstairs, I find his office and a waiting room with three chairs. I am anxious to the bones, jiggling my foot up and down, forwards and back, around and around. There's something about seeing a psychiatrist that feels particularly shameful. I keep my head bowed down as his previous patient walks past me. I do not want to be seen. I do not want to be recognised.

'Ariane? Come on in.' The psychiatrist is a man in his fifties with grey hair and photos of his teenage daughters on his desk. I scan the books on the shelves behind him and take a deep breath.

In the weeks before this first appointment, for reasons I still do not understand, I become fixated on Charmaine Dragun. Dragun, a Channel Ten newsreader, took her own life when she was just twenty-nine years old. At the time of her death, Robb also worked at Ten in a small digital media team. We are physically similar – small with brown hair and brown eyes. I am twenty-eight years old.

I read the coroner's report, which was released in October 2010, while Henry naps. I'm so tired that sometimes I read it with one eye closed. We both experienced disordered eating, we are both perfectionists, and her 'highs' and 'lows' echo my own. Soon I know parts of it by heart:

She was ... [v]ery effervescent and it struck me as a little bit unusual ... sometimes within an hour she'd be very up and then sort of come down quite quickly.

She would bounce into the room, jumping up and down.

She wouldn't just hug you, she would squeeze you.

When I bring her up, the psychiatrist doesn't want to talk about Charmaine: 'Why are you reading that?' Instead, he wants to talk about my mother and asks me if I've considered going into hospital.

'You're a psychologist,' he says, looking at my referral. 'Have you tried any cognitive or behavioural techniques?'

You're a psychologist, I hear. *Why haven't you been able to fix yourself?*

He prints off a Black Dog Institute chart for bipolar disorder, saying, 'There's an emerging literature around mothers and first episode bipolar type 2.' I feel the heat swell in my cheeks, and think of the scene in the film *The Virgin Suicides* where the youngest Lisbon sister asks her doctor, 'What would you know about being a teenage girl?' I want to say to the psychiatrist, 'What the fuck could you possibly know about being a new mum? How the fuck could you possibly help me?' But I don't. Instead, I pay for the session and leave.

I don't tell him that I can't see the baby's face properly, that there's something wrong with him, and that I don't know how to bond with what I can't see. I don't tell him that sometimes the baby turns into a dragon – just a flash and then it's gone. I don't tell him that I know DoCS will remove the baby because of his terrible nappy rash – that it's only a matter of time. That I have seen this happen; I have done this to other mothers. That I am scared it's DoCS every time there's a knock on the door. I don't tell him that I am starting to see death everywhere, that I'm not sure if I exist. That I think I might already be dead. That I wonder if I might end up like Charmaine. I don't tell him, I don't tell him, I don't tell him. Because what if he reports me to the board and says I'm too broken to ever practise? What then?

⳾

I am constantly being asked, 'Why didn't anyone know? How did you go under the radar for so long with something so serious?' But I'm not alone in this. I find an article written by psychiatrist Professor Marie-Paule Austin in *O&G Magazine* about the difficulty of detecting postpartum psychosis in milder cases, where symptoms can be minimised or where women have some insight. 'These women may present well at cross-sectional assessment,' she writes, noting that it's important to speak to significant others and to review the woman at regular and close intervals.

'More subtle forms of psychosis are going to be picked up later,' agrees Dr Katherine Wisner, a professor of psychiatry and obstetrics, in an interview with *The New York Times*. 'These women tend to have prolonged delusional thinking: "there's something really wrong with my baby".'

I was *these* women. I presented well. I was not well.

'You'd cover the pram with those muslin wraps,' Robb says. 'You always had him covered up. You were always hiding him from other people. I just thought you were worried about the sun. If I'd had any idea how sick you were, I'd never have got on those planes.'

⳾

In a group chat, my siblings and I compare war stories about our father – practically a celebrity doctor in the suburb we grew up in – being utterly unimpressed with any medical condition we brought to him. Classic kids-of-a-GP stuff.

'My tonsils,' Lulu says. 'Took years to get those fuckers out.'

'Giardia,' I say. 'That time I had giardia and looked emaciated. Dad finally dug out some Flagyl. Sweet relief.'

'My ankle,' Huw says. 'Practically broken but "just let it heal".'

'Migraines,' Evan adds. '"You'll grow out of it." Absolutely not bothered.'

'Good one,' I say.

'I've just found all my old school reports,' Evan texts back, 'and my attendance is nearly flawless because you could not get away with a Bueller-style sick day. He was Dr House MD before it was cool (and it was absolutely fucking not lupus).'

'The grandkids though,' I text. 'They practically get an inter-disciplinary case conference every time their temperature hits 37.4 degrees.'

∾

Robb's mum, Penny, flies down from Brisbane while Milly is in respite care to look after the baby so that Robb and I can have a night away. Penny takes him to her hotel as we drive to the Blue Mountains. She sends us photos of the baby in a fluffy white towel, grinning on her double bed.

He looks so happy with her.

'I think I miss him,' I tell Robb later that night. 'I guess that's a good sign?'

After we get home, I escape to the local shopping centre. I walk down through the park, music screaming in my ears. I am alone; I am still tethered to the baby.

Inside the centre, I march through the busy food court, trying to focus on what I came for. I need clothes. My maternity wardrobe is too big, and my pre-baby clothing feels all wrong. I am not that girl anymore.

I drift from shop to shop, not finding anything. The rows of clothes are intimidating. There is too much choice. Was there always this much choice?

A mannequin from Cotton On waves at me as I walk past, turns her head to watch me go.

What's the point of buying clothes when you're not going to be around for much longer? says a voice in my head.

The thought is oddly comforting. I have a way out. At the top of the escalators, I imagine myself falling, falling, all the way to the bottom.

Not today, I think, *but soon. Soon.*

ᔎ

'How did you feel after our last session?' the psychiatrist asks me during our second appointment a week later.

'Worse,' I tell him. 'I wanted to throw myself off the escalators at Broadway.'

'Oh,' he says, looking at his notes. 'What did we talk about last time?'

I tell Dr Wilson that I'm not going back.

ᔎ

'Arns!' I wake to Robb yelling my name and cursing the gods. Henry is crying in his cot.

'What's wrong?' I yell back, checking my phone. It's after two a.m.

I scoop Henry up and run downstairs to where Robb is grabbing buckets and towels. Part of the ceiling in our living room has collapsed and rain is streaming through. There's water everywhere. The wind howls.

Henry screams in his bouncer next to us while I replace one soaked towel after another, wringing them out in the sink and laying them down again.

The rain eventually stops. The wind keeps howling.

∽

I am convinced the baby doesn't like me. I am not bonding with him, and he isn't developing an attachment to me either. He is better off without me. Everyone is better off without me.

He is better off without me. Everyone is better off without me. He is better off without me. Everyone is better off without me.

Without me, without me, without me.

Ruminate: from the Latin *ruminatus*, past participle of *ruminare*, 'to chew the cud'.

∽

The baby looks up at me from his pram and squeals.

Just walk into the traffic.

We are standing at the lights of a busy inner-city intersection, waiting to cross the road. The pram wheels are on the ramp, primed. Traffic is tearing past and I clasp the handle. My fingernails leave crescents in both palms.

Robb appears then, through the doors of the bottle shop.

I grab the wine from his hands and push the pram in his direction.

'You need to take him,' I say.

'Are you okay?' he asks.

'No.'

When we get home, I tell Robb I am going for a walk. The truth is, I want to run. I want to peel away my skin, step out of this body, this mind I do not recognise and start over again somewhere else. I wonder if I am going mad or if, perhaps, I am simply a monster. A psychopath. Is one better than the other?

But I do not run. Instead, I pace around the back streets of Redfern.

I remember the sky was sprinkled with stars.

I remember the throb of my heart.

I remember the tears so hot they felt like glass.

And then the bough breaks, and you fall, fall, fall to the floor of yourself.

∽

'I think you need to go into hospital,' says Dr Wilson. The silence between us is so fragile I'm scared to speak in case it shatters.

Henry, crawling at my feet, starts to grizzle, and I rummage in my handbag for one of his toys.

'Hope the floor's clean,' I say with a sigh, watching as he drops his rusk then puts it straight back into his mouth.

'The floor's fine, Ariane,' Dr Wilson says softly. He turns his chair back to his computer and types. 'You're not getting better. Your depression is severe. We need to try a new medication and I just don't know how quickly I can get you in to see someone else. The psychiatrist came highly recommended but we don't always get it right first go. There's a great female psychologist I'd refer you to, but she's on leave for the next few weeks.'

'I don't know if I can start again with someone else. It takes too long.'

'I know.'

Eyes filling and overflowing, I try to process Dr Wilson's words. They are coming out too fast. He's now on the phone to hospital admissions, rattling off my name and age. The woman he's describing doesn't sound like me at all.

'How old is Henry?' he asks me.

'Nine months.'

'He's nine months,' Dr Wilson says to the admissions office. 'Okay, thank you.'

'Right,' he says, hanging up the phone. 'They have a bed for you. Obviously, it's Good Friday tomorrow and I don't think there's much use you being there over Easter. What about we admit you Tuesday morning? Do you think you can wait until then?'

I look at my shoes, bright red ballet flats, then back up at him.

'I think it's the right decision,' he says, reading my mind.

'Yeah?'

'Yes. At least in hospital you can taper off the Zoloft and they'll try you on something else. And you'll meet other women going through what you're experiencing, too.'

'Okay.'

'I'll call them back and let them know.'

I phone my dad on the way home and burst into tears when he answers.

'Arnie?'

'They want me to go into hospital.'

'Which one?

'St John of God. They take mums and babies?'

'Burwood. Yes. Are you safe?'

'Yes. I'm just walking Henry home.'

'I'll be right over.'

I feel something I haven't felt in a long time: I just want my dad.

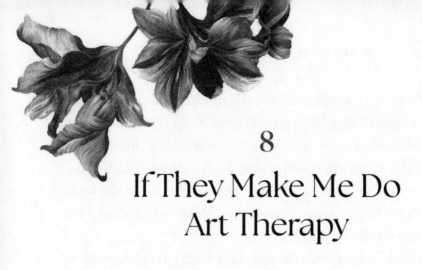

8
If They Make Me Do Art Therapy

Inpatient *(noun): a person who stays in hospital*
for medical treatment.
Impatient *(adjective): wanting something to happen*
as soon as possible.

'If they make me do art therapy, I'm leaving,' I tell Robb. We are in the car, on our way to the mother and baby psychiatric unit in St John of God Hospital, Burwood.

'You'll be fine,' Robb says, laughing, but I can tell he's nervous too.

Mother and baby units (or MBUs) are a special type of hospital care for women with severe perinatal mental illness. Staffed by psychiatrists, social workers and psychologists, MBUs allow mums to be treated with their babies, rather than separating them during a period that is critical for bonding and attachment. At the time, it was the only unit of its kind in NSW – and it was in a private hospital. I am fortunate, privileged. Not only do I have private health insurance, but there's a bed available and the ward is about twenty minutes away from home.

In the lead-up to my admission, during the four blurry days

of the Easter long weekend, I have felt strangely calm, even questioning whether I should go into hospital. Surely there are others who need the bed more than me? But as we drive along Parramatta Road in the afternoon traffic, I am overcome with tears. I turn my face away from the baby, who is oblivious in the back seat, with his bright green dinosaur toy. Robb puts his hand on mine, concentrates on the road.

At the admissions office the tears keep falling. It's embarrassing how little control I have over them. I swat them away and they stain the endless forms I'm required to fill out: the Edinburgh Postnatal Depression Scale, the Depression, Anxiety and Stress Scale and attachment and bonding measures. There are so many questions.

The kind woman behind the desk hands me a wad of tissues and says, apologetically, that she needs to take a photo of me. And so I look straight down into the barrel of the camera and smile, a broad, wet, incongruous smile, because that's what I've always done; I smile. She prints the photo, black and white, and affixes it to my file.

I hand over my Zoloft, the medication I'm to be tapered off. It has made me worse, not better. They'll dole out the little white pills now, in increasingly small doses, until it's out of my system.

'The nurses will check on you every hour for the first day,' the woman says. 'You can't leave the grounds without permission, not until you're cleared to a lower security level. And when you do have permission, you'll have to sign in and out on the board and say where you're going. I'll show you where that is.'

Staying in this hospital is voluntary and I can leave at any time – but the rules feel scary and real.

'Do you have any questions?' the woman asks.

'Not yet,' I say. 'Thank you.'

'Alright, let me buzz someone from the unit.'

Robb smiles at me from behind a wiggly baby.

'Ariane?' A nurse pokes her head around the office door.

'Yeah.'

'How about I show you to your room?'

∽

Unsurprisingly, perhaps, this part is hard to write. As I sit in front of my laptop and try to find the words, I am simultaneously standing on the threshold of that unit, at the head of the long corridor lined with patients' rooms. My stomach is a closed fist. Even now there is shame. Even now there is guilt that my son's first year of life involved a psychiatric ward. Shall we walk down the corridor together? Shall we open the door to this room I've kept closed for many years now?

I think it's time.

∽

The consultant psychiatrist assigned to me for the duration of my stay has thick black glasses and speaks in a low monotone. I'm to see her briefly twice a week – on Tuesdays and Fridays. Her registrar is a man, about thirty, with floppy dark hair. He's dressed in suit pants and a blue shirt and reminds me of Zach Braff.

I don't remember much of that first meeting, but Robb does. 'You went into clinical mode,' he says. 'It was strange to watch. You were aggressive. Blunt. Rude. And you were lying to them. You were underselling how bad it was.'

'Really?'

'Yes! I kept thinking, *She can't treat you if she doesn't know what's going on.* But when I tried to intervene or correct you, I felt as though they didn't want me around. Remember, she said, "Why don't you wait outside with Henry?" I felt stunned. Neither of them spoke to me. I remember standing outside in the corridor with a crying baby, while my wife was in the room just lying to the doctors. I thought, *These guys don't know what they're doing.*'

What I do remember is one exchange before Robb left the room with Henry. The psychiatrist is saying she'll take me off Zoloft and try me on mirtazapine, a tetracyclic or atypical antidepressant.

'Now, it's likely that you'll gain about three or four kilos on this medication,' she says, looking down at my file. 'Is that okay?'

'Sure,' I say. 'No problems.'

Robb turns to face me and raises an eyebrow, but doesn't say anything.

Not a chance, I think.

⁓

The first night on the ward, I lie awake listening to a newborn crying in the room next door. The sound hurts my skull. Our room has a double bed, a bathroom and a white cot tucked under the window.

As part of the admission, you can opt for the nurses to take your baby for the first two nights. This is a period of consolidated rest – something many women need urgently. But now that I am no longer 'starving him' and he is completely formula-fed, Henry is chubby and happy and healthy and sleeps through most of the night. He snores softly in his blue teddy-bear sleep suit.

Robb texts to say he loves us both and that he'll be back tomorrow. It's too far for him to commute each day to work, so we agree he'll stay at home and visit us each night instead of sleeping here, like some of the other families do.

Wide awake, I unfriend several Facebook friends. I do not want anyone watching me while I'm in here. I still can't sleep – my body has forgotten how.

In my suitcase I packed a book about motherhood edited by Jessica Rowe. But I am not in any of its pages. There are no mental health professionals who can't seem to remember how to stay alive. There are no women on psychiatric wards.

I don't know how I got here, I write in a new journal. I have always written my way through difficult periods of my life. In my wardrobe there's a box full of journals I kept through high school and university.

In hospital, though, they're the only words I'll write.

∽

The next morning, the ward manager introduces me to some of the other mums and their babies in the unit meeting. There's one of these meetings each day at nine a.m. and I'm told we must get dressed for them – no pyjamas, no slippers. I wear jeans and a jumper and smear foundation on my face.

Henry is the eldest baby by some months and the most mobile. While we're going around the circle sharing our names, he lifts himself up and knocks a stack of magazines onto the floor with a thud and a grin.

'Oh god, that looks exhausting,' says Fiona, one of the mums, as she watches Henry crawl away from the magazines. Her baby, a newborn with thick, dark hair, is fast asleep in her arms.

'It is,' I sigh, scooping Henry up.

As we file out of the room, one of the counsellors asks me, 'How are you feeling, Ariane?' I tell her that I don't think I can stay here / I'm not sure it's for me / not sure it's the 'right fit' / not sure I'm bad enough / I'm a psychologist, see / I'm not sure I'm going to stay / just not sure it's for me.

She smiles kindly, says my reaction is quite normal and suggests I give it a little longer. 'You know,' she says, wiping the whiteboard clean and following me out into the corridor. 'Most mothers don't want to leave.'

In her book *Small Acts of Disappearance,* Fiona Wright recalls being admitted to an eating disorders unit in Sydney for treatment for anorexia nervosa. 'I still remember thinking, even then, that I'd have nothing in common at all with any of the other women I might meet there. Because I wasn't, I thought, one of those women,' she writes. And yet, as Wright soon discovers, 'I couldn't help but recognise myself reflected in the stories they told.'

Even then, I didn't believe I was unwell. I wasn't as sick as *those* mothers. I didn't really belong there.

∽

In the nursery where I make Henry's bottles, I find an art therapy class timetable affixed to the wall. I snap a photo and send it to Robb.

Monday 12 p.m.–1 p.m.
Tuesday 12 p.m.–1 p.m.
Wednesday 12 p.m.–1 p.m.
Thursday 12 p.m.–1 p.m.
Friday 12 p.m.–1 p.m.
Weekends CLOSED

'Every fucking day,' I text him. 'See? Exactly what I thought.'

'Arns,' he replies, 'that's the time the art room is *open*. Not when you need to be in there.'

'Still.'

'I'll see you both later. Be there around six.'

∽

I meet Carolyn and her baby, Jackson, in the nursery on my first morning. She's dressed in jeans and a t-shirt and is mixing a bottle – boiling water, scooping formula, stirring.

'How old is Jackson?' I ask.

'Seven months,' she says, smiling while putting the lid back on the tin of formula. 'And Henry?'

'Nine months,' I say, watching as she clasps a bib onto Jackson and hands him the bottle. There's an efficiency about her movements – a competence that seems out of place.

'Did you just get here?' she asks.

'Yesterday, yeah. You?'

'I came in before Easter,' Carolyn says. 'Which wasn't great because no one was here all weekend.' She laughs. 'It was pretty quiet.'

I watch as Henry crawls towards a pile of toys left on the nursery floor.

'Everyone else's babies are so much younger,' I say. 'Like newborns.'

'Yeah,' Carolyn says. 'I found that hard too.'

We're silent for a moment, both understanding what the other is thinking: we've been sad for too long now.

It hurts.

∽

At ten a.m. and two p.m. (sharp) each weekday, we have compulsory group therapy. Before each session, we drop the babies off at the nursery to be looked after for the hour, then sit in a circle with one of the unit staff. Some of the courses are run by psychologists, some by nurses, some by the unit psychiatrists.

I still have my workbook from those sessions (*No swearing!* reads one of the group rules), despite the content being comically dated in parts, highly gendered and heteronormative. It's full of cognitive behaviour therapy (CBT) techniques and mindfulness exercises. There's a 'stress bucket' I've diligently filled out, 'bad day' plans and lists of the 'Myths of Motherhood':

Motherhood is a woman's ultimate life fulfillment.
A mother instantly feels love and attachment to her baby.
A woman has motherly instincts, so she knows how to be a mother.
Breast is always best.

Next to 'Breastfeeding is easy and doesn't hurt,' I've scribbled in red pen: 'Mum BF all four of us.'

There's an exercise we must have completed as a group, capturing our thoughts during times of stress. On a blank page I've written:

Baby not sleeping

Not tonight, not again.
I can never settle you.
Nothing works.
What's wrong with you?
I can't do this.
I'm hopeless.

I didn't want this.

I'm so tired.

Breastfeeding not working

Why can't I do this?

Everyone else can do this.

Is he getting enough?

Why won't you eat?

Just eat.

What else can I do?

Maybe it would be easier to bottle feed.

But I don't want to bottle feed.

I'm a failure.

I'm hopeless.

Why is he rejecting me?

I've tried everything.

∽

I am walking through the local shopping centre after restocking Henry's favourite food pouches when the ground beneath me shakes. My first thought is that I have tripped over something, but then it happens again, this time more intensely. I feel the jolt under my feet, all the way through to my fingertips. As I push the pram past the shops, the music is suddenly too loud. The harsh fluorescent lights hurt my eyes. The panic rises in my chest. I make it back to hospital, the little jolts a heartbeat in my shoes.

That afternoon during group therapy, I ask the pharmacist, 'How long will the brain shocks last?' It's his turn to deliver a session, this time about medication and possible side effects. For most of us, it's the first time we've been prescribed psychiatric medication.

'Brain shocks?' he says. 'You mean ECT?'

'No, no,' I say, 'not ECT. The withdrawal shocks. From the Zoloft.'

'Oh, I see,' he says. 'I'm not too sure. It can vary. Have you mentioned that to your psychiatrist?'

After the session, Zach Braff is summonsed by one of the nurses. I am sitting cross-legged on my bed while Henry plays in his cot next to me. Zach seems nervous.

'What are the tears about?' he asks.

I stare at him in disbelief. *I'm a psychologist in a psychiatric ward. My entire world has been turned upside down. I feel nothing towards my baby. Haven't I ticked that box? The baby doesn't even like me. I'm too unwell to go back to work. What are the fucking tears about?*

Of course, I don't say any of that. Instead, I mumble something about feeling electric shocks through my entire body, that they're so strong they jolt me when I walk and how long are they likely to last, please?

Zach, unsurprisingly, can't tell me – at least not with the precision I need to hear. What he can tell me is that the jolts are known as 'discontinuation syndrome', an array of symptoms one experiences when withdrawing or tapering from antidepressants.

When I go searching for information about brain zaps, what's interesting is the subjectivity of how they're experienced. In one paper they're described as a 'jolt sensation', 'like seizures', 'brain reboot blinks', 'orgasm, but irritating', 'orgasm, but not in a good way'.

No one, it seems, can say how long they'll last.

As the Zoloft leaves my system, I become flushed with rage. Fury. I sign myself out of hospital to let staff know I've gone for a walk and do laps of the park with the pram while Sia's 'Wild

Ones' blares in my ears. The weather is getting colder as we rush towards winter and the wind lashes my cheeks.

Henry chews on a purple pouch of baby food, grins up at me with Robb's blue eyes.

I walk and walk, around and around, until it gets dark.

In *Nightbitch*, Rachel Yoder writes, 'Yes, certainly, her emerging rage was in part a by-product of physiological processes, but how could you not be pissed after having a baby?'

How could you not? I am feral with rage.

My anger changes shape. It fixes on the patients in the cafeteria from other wards. They swarm around Henry when I'm trying to feed him or trying to eat something myself. I feel on show when I only want to disappear.

'Isn't he a cutie?'

'How ya going, mum?'

'What are you eating today, bud? Eat your veggies.'

These intrusions, always well intentioned, make me irrationally angry. I want to scream, *Leave me alone!* But I don't. I swallow the screams one by one, with the mushy peas and the mashed potatoes, and vow not to eat there again.

Robb lugs Henry's highchair from home into hospital then sets it up in our room. I bring our meals down from the cafeteria and we eat in peace, alone.

∽

The Circle of Security, the 'visual map of attachment' I taped to my office wall at DoCS, appears again, this time during group therapy one morning. The group leader talks us through the guiding idea behind the circle – that as parents we are both a secure base and a safe haven for our children. We are there, watching and delighting, as they explore the world, and we are there to comfort them when they return.

Always be
BIGGER, STRONGER, WISER AND KIND.
Whenever possible
FOLLOW MY CHILD'S LEAD.
Wherever necessary
TAKE CHARGE.

'Always be' feels like an impossible command. I am not the bigger, stronger, wiser or kind parent I thought I would be, the one I'd teach foster parents about in my old life as they tried to understand the little ones in their care. This time, I am on the other side – it's *my* circle, *my* baby – and I'm the one who needs help.

Watch over me
Delight in me
Help me
Enjoy with me.

Help me.

ᔐ

'Do you remember much about when I was filmed?' I ask Robb.

'Yeah.' He practically snorts. 'Do I ever. You were absolutely filthy about it.'

After group therapy one morning, a nurse knocks on my door. 'Do you have a moment?' she asks. 'I thought it might be a good time to do your filming.'

I groan. I do not want to be watched. I know what they're doing.

In the patient manual, I had read about this 'unique aspect' of the program, where each mother is filmed interacting with her baby: 'You could be doing just about any activity – playing on a rug, giving your baby a bath, reading to your baby – whatever activity you feel more comfortable doing.' The point is to highlight a positive mothering experience and 'to learn more about the special ways in which you and your baby are beginning to get to know each other'.

I nod to the nurse, lift Henry and follow her into the nursery. It's a small room full of second-hand toys and a wooden rocking chair. There's a bright foam play mat on the floor. While she sets up the camera and tripod, I find a book and a set of blocks.

'Alright then,' she says, smiling. 'Whenever you're ready.'

It's hard to describe the shame of this moment, or why this scene in my mind feels like the definition of rock bottom. It isn't, of course – not even close. Rock bottom, whatever that means, was yet to come. But the act of being watched, of being the observed, not the observer, of being on the other side of the camera, is one I won't, I can't, forget.

Have you ever watched a ballet dancer and wondered how they make something so difficult look so easy? From our first class, we're taught how to perform – to project, to spin and balance and jump – without the effort of these movements showing on our face. As Susan Sontag writes, 'The dancer's performance smile is not so much a smile as simply a categorical denial of what he or she is actually experiencing.' Effort lives in the muscles, the tendons and the hours of repetition in studios, failing and failing better. To show exertion is to reveal what's behind the curtain.

How much of these moments of early motherhood were performance? For years I'd learnt how to dance in pain, blistered toes bleeding into the shank of my pointe shoe; to hold a 'pleasant expression' while standing on one leg in a corps de ballet. Is it any wonder I could perform scenes of motherhood, perfectly, on command?

When the filming is over, the nurse packs away the equipment and says, 'You're beautiful with him.' I have held it together up until now, camera-ready for my performance. But her words make me burst into tears.

'Thank you,' I say. 'But it's taking everything I've got. And I've got nothing left.'

ς

I first hear about the Tronick still face experiment years later, at the Childbirth and Parenting Educators conference on the Sunshine Coast. The experiment, developed in the 1970s by Edward Tronick, begins with a mum and her baby interacting face to face. They smile, make eye contact, giggle. After this initial interaction, the still face condition begins. Mum looks away from her baby then turns back to him, expressionless, emotionless and unresponsive for three minutes.

The baby points, smiles, puts his hands up. He then screeches, becomes floppy, cries – anything to bring mum 'back'. As Tronick writes:

He makes repeated attempts to get the interaction into its usual reciprocal pattern. When these attempts fail, the infant withdraws [and] orients his face and body away from his mother with a withdrawn, hopeless facial expression.

Videos of the experiment are distressing to watch – not least because the mother's lack of expression in the still face condition mirrors what a depressive episode can look like. And as we know – as I know – these can last a lot longer than three minutes. It's hard not to worry about the damage I might have done, about the short- and long-term impacts of maternal depression when the research is this stark. I scroll paper after paper online.

> We present a model that in part accounts for the toxic effects of maternal depression on a child's social–emotional functioning and development.

There's only so much my heart can take.
I log off.

How do we measure love? That question again – different though, now, from those early, hormone-soaked hours after the birth. Of course, it's not really love we're measuring or looking for in these observations, but rather attachment – the nature of the relationship between parent and baby.

'There's no baby without a mother,' paediatrician and psychoanalyst D.W. Winnicott once said. There is no baby without a mother.

I am thinking now of what it means to be watched, under surveillance, judged. For all the hospital's soft language, I understood that in that nursery I was being observed, so that my interactions, attachment and mothering skills could all be assessed.

I am thinking of the first time I supervised a contact visit as a caseworker, the way I sat in the small room, making notes. The mother was young and during the visit she fed and changed her baby. Had I ever fed or changed a baby? I'm embarrassed to admit that I don't think I had – yet there I was, compiling notes, evidence for the court, and no doubt casting judgement.

I am thinking of when I was a provisional psychologist, sitting at the back of a McDonald's in south-west Sydney, shadowing my colleague's assessment. The little girl had been in out-of-home care for two years and we were observing one of her six annual scheduled visits with her family. We got there before the family arrived and ordered coffees. 'Lara's been having some trouble at school,' my colleague told me, 'and at home now, too.' We planned to do a general needs assessment – an IQ test using the WISC (Wechsler Intelligence Scale for Children) behaviour checklist, interviews with her teachers and foster carers and observations at school, at home and during contact visits.

'The foster carers are worried because her behaviour always gets worse after seeing mum and dad,' my colleague told me, reading through his notes. 'Which is quite normal. So we'll just see how it goes.'

It was a different sort of visit – instead of supervising, which the allocated caseworker did, we sat and observed. Lara and her siblings arrived in their school uniforms, took the presents their parents brought with them and climbed over the play equipment outside.

The visit was only two hours long and Lara cried when it was time to leave. I made a note of this in my file. What else was there to say?

⁓

'You're a professional, too?' Fiona asks me one morning as we're waiting for coffee at the hospital coffee cart. She and her eight-week-old baby are admitted about a week after me.

'A psychologist, yeah,' I say. 'Well, I mean I was. I guess. How about you?'

'I'm a dentist,' she says. 'I mean, well, same. I was.'

Fiona is pale and wears oversized shirts and fluffy slippers. Her eyes are lined with dark circles. She is utterly shocked by motherhood – but, unlike me, she doesn't for one second pretend not to be. It has taken me years to recognise how brave this is.

We take our coffees back to where group therapy is about to start, via the nursery where we leave our babies. As I peel Henry from where he's curled around my hip, he starts to cry and reaches out for me.

'Oh gosh, I find that so heartbreaking,' Fiona says, as she watches me place him on the ground and find his new favourite truck. But I am not heartbroken. Instead, his little protest makes me smile – it means he doesn't want me to go, doesn't want me to leave him. Perhaps he likes me after all?

'I'll be back soon, baby,' I tell Henry, handing him to one of the nurses.

'We've got him,' she says, smiling.

'Thank you.'

My heart swells and swells and swells.

Henry's reaction makes me think of Mary Ainsworth's Strange Situation Procedure, which was developed in 1969 to understand attachment styles between mothers and babies. In the procedure, babies experience two brief separations from their mother and two reunions, in an unfamiliar playroom and with the introduction of a stranger. The brief separations are designed to increase the baby's stress, to observe how they respond. As you might imagine, babies react slightly differently but in predictable patterns to the anxiety of the separations, the presence of the stranger and the subsequent reunions with their caregiver.

In their classic text *Patterns of Attachment*, Ainsworth and her co-authors explain that it's the *reunion* episodes, where mum re-joins baby after a few minutes away, that are the most significant, not the separations. The way a baby approaches their caregiver at this moment – whether they seek comfort, are angry or avoid contact – determines whether they're classified as secure (B), insecure avoidant (A) or insecure ambivalent/resistant (C). A fourth style – disorganised attachment (D), where babies exhibit 'odd' and 'inexplicable' behaviour – came with later research by Main and Solomon.

The Strange Situation was designed for research purposes, not clinical assessment, and is not without criticism. Some of this relates to the way it has been and continues to be applied in the child protection system, especially to justify child removal. Yet its underlying concepts provide a framework for understanding the parent–infant relationship and how this might be disrupted in the context of perinatal mental illness. It's also why keeping mothers and babies together, such as in mother and baby units, where it's safe to do so, is considered best practice when treating these conditions.

After group therapy, I walk back to the nursery with the other mums. Henry is on the floor playing, but when he sees me he smiles, squeals and starts crawling towards the baby gate. I pick him up and kiss him on the cheek.

Reunited.

My heart swells again – the balm of it.

Although my love for Henry grows stronger, I never really settle into life on the mother and baby ward, at least not in the way other mothers seem to. Yet it's a relief not to have to worry about cooking and cleaning (or not cooking and not cleaning), to just focus on recovering and on bonding with Henry. I feel protected from the world, from the everyday noise of living I had become too porous to filter out.

I learn what it means to be assessed, analysed and asked the same questions over and over again. I feel, keenly, how re-traumatising and depleting it can be to repeat your story for different clinicians, the way they all probe in slightly different ways and zero in on different things. The way you can start to question your own memory, your own symptoms, your own experience. I think about the way I've spoken to parents in the past, the times when I went over and over the same details. I am tired of my own voice. I am tired of my own story.

I am tired.

∽

Ballet is synonymous with perfection – with line, placement, precision. 'Perfect practice makes perfect,' my Russian ballet teacher used to say to us. She wore green parachute pants and was so thin you could count the bones in her chest.

Ribs in.

Shoulders down.

Knees back.

Heels forward.

Eyes up.

We all knew that no matter how hard we practised, we would never be perfect. But that didn't mean we stopped trying.

I was introduced to the concept of the 'good-enough mother' during my early training as a caseworker. In the context of child protection work, a good-enough mother was one who met the basic non-negotiables when it came to parenting capacity. For this reason, in my mind, being 'good enough' seemed a pejorative statement – the very least we were able to 'accept'.

Perhaps unsurprisingly, there's a strong association between perfectionism and perinatal mental health problems. Yet the idea of the good-enough mother, coined by Winnicott in 1951, relies on imperfection. 'The good-enough mother … starts off with an almost complete adaptation to her infant's needs, and as time proceeds, she adapts less and less completely, gradually, according to the infant's growing ability to deal with her failure.'

In other words, not being a perfect parent teaches our babies about the imperfect world they've been born into. And by not being perfect, we let our children know they don't need to be perfect either.

⟳

'You *did* present well,' my aunt Glyn texts me. She and my other aunty, Meri, visited me while I was on the ward. 'I remember that. You were trying so hard to be "normal" and looking after Henry. It was as though you were a shell – there in body but the "you" was missing. Your body looked sad. As a dancer you were always so confident and held yourself so well. But my lasting impression of you in that room was of a shell. Sad. Lifeless, almost. I cried when we left.'

⟳

In group therapy one morning, the psychologist places laminated black-and-white photos on the floor. They are photos of objects such as prams and bottles, as well as more abstract images and patterns – a modern Rorschach of sorts. She asks us to choose one and share part of our story. I hold up my photo. It's of a woman sitting with an older lady, who is cradling her baby.

'My mum still works pretty much full-time, teaching. And I have three siblings but they're all younger than me and none of them have kids. My youngest brother is only twenty-one. And my dad works full-time too. He's a doctor. And my in-laws are in Brisbane. And I'm the first of any of my friends to have a baby so no one knows how to help, even though my friend Brooke has tried. And my friend Jo moved to Canberra and my friend Paul went overseas to do a PhD. And my best friend Lizzie has chronic health problems at the moment, so I don't like to bother her too much. And Robb, my husband, travelled quite a bit for work. So, I was on my own a lot.'

'That must have been really hard,' the psychologist says.

'Oh, it was fine,' I say with a shrug. 'You know how it is.'

'That must have been really hard,' she says again.

∾

I don't take many photos of my own while on the ward. There's a few of Henry in his cot, smiling, always smiling. But there is one that pops up in my Facebook memories each year. Evan visits one evening, bringing food and books and toys for Henry. The two of them play in the nursery while I have a shower.

Later that night, when I go back to the nursery to heat up a bottle for Henry, I see the giant nursery bear, a bear the size of me, reading a copy of *Twilight* in the wooden rocking chair. I know it's Evan's handiwork and it makes me laugh for the first time in what feels like weeks.

I tell the next doctor about Evan during our session the following day – about how close we've always been and how much

135

he adores Henry. She's yet another psychiatrist, another notepad, another pen, another beige clinic room. This one, unlike the one I met initially, is supposed to do more intensive therapeutic work, rather than just an assessment and a medication review. She is young and thoughtful and calming and asks me about my family and my work before my symptoms.

'Now, when you say Henry looked strange,' she says, glancing at her notes, 'what exactly did you mean?'

The question takes me by surprise. No one else has probed this far. Did I really let that slip? But as I gather my thoughts, there's a knock on the door – like in a scene from a film.

'Excuse me just a moment,' the doctor says.

The timing is comedic. Did she step out of the room to talk to the person who was looking for her? Or did she just stand at the door? I don't remember. But I do remember her coming back and asking me something else.

The moment is lost. I do not help her find it.

∽

While our stories, our backgrounds and our symptoms are all different, there's one thread common to all the mums on the ward with me – a sense of shame that we are there, that we need help. My own shame is multilayered – I am a mental health professional with a mental illness. Have I, by speaking up, ruined my career just as it is getting off the ground? Will I ever be well enough to work again?

It was Carl Jung who first described the concept of the 'Wounded Healer'. 'It is [your] own hurt which gives the measure of [your] power to heal,' he wrote back in 1951. But while it's almost a cliché that many enter helping professions to understand their

136

own struggles, that doesn't mean it's at all acceptable. In 2022, an article in *The Conversation* noted that: 'Psychologists are just starting to talk publicly about their own mental illness.' *Just.* New research into the rate of mental health conditions among applied psychologists found that in the group of 1692 respondents, more than 80 per cent reported a history of mental health difficulties, while nearly half had received a mental health diagnosis. The study also acknowledged that information about 'this question is para-doxically neglected, perhaps because disclosure and discussion of these experiences remain taboo within the field'.

One of my favourite and most returned-to memoirs is Kay Redfield Jamison's *An Unquiet Mind*. In it, the professor of psy-chiatry shared her concerns around being honest about her bipolar disorder. 'Whatever the consequences, they are bound to be better than continuing to be silent. I am tired of hiding, tired of misspent and knotted energies, tired of the hypocrisy, and tired of acting as though I have something to hide.'

It will take several years before I'll feel the same way.

A memory. I am on the nightshift at Lifeline one Saturday. I only do nights on weekends because staying awake from ten p.m. until six a.m. knocks my sleep cycle around so much it takes me days to recover. Between calls, I study for my end-of-year exams – statis-tics and abnormal psychology. It's my last set of exams before I graduate.

I take a call around midnight. It's an older man who seems lonely more than anything else.

'Your voice sounds like a little bird,' he says. 'I'm going to call you Little Bird.'

The man tells me he was a clinical psychologist many years ago – and has since retired.

'Only already broken people go into psychotherapy, Little Bird,' he says. 'You sound nice. Young, but nice. But you should think about why you're doing this.'

I don't think I've ever stopped thinking about it.

⌇

One of the MBU's rules is that we are not to enter another patient's room or exchange contact details. From the manual again: 'It is important to focus on your own recovery and not to be involved in others' recovery. We strongly discourage you being in contact with others outside of the group. Other group members are NOT a part of your support network. They are only your support inside the group.'

'What do you remember about that time?' I ask Carolyn recently. We are still close friends and are celebrating our kids' tenth birthdays. The boys run around a noisy arcade while Robb and I sip wine with Carolyn and her husband, Si.

'Well, I remember you didn't give a shit about the rules,' she chuckles.

As patients, Carolyn and I spend hours doing loops of the park outside the hospital with our prams, trying to figure out why our brains no longer work the way they used to. We learn about one another's lives over terrible hospital coffee and in the group therapy that rips us open every morning and attempts to stitch us back together.

Carolyn is insightful and clever and funny. She tells me about her parents – her mother has schizophrenia and her father has bipolar disorder – and how so much of her life has been spent caring for them. For Carolyn, the anxiety after Jackson was born has been deeply physical. It's in her wrists – a tingling sensation. Sometimes, it's a current that runs through her entire body.

In her presence, however, I only feel calm.

Carolyn and I do a yoga class, off-loading our babies onto the nurses beforehand and giggling, as if we're headed to a girls' night out. The class is upstairs in one of the rooms attached to the mood disorders unit and mostly full of patients we haven't met. Some of their faces are familiar from the cafeteria.

I unroll a yoga mat, lift my leg to the ceiling and point my toe. The body remembers – my muscles creak into their familiar places.

The woman beside us farts through every position, announcing each new pose. Carolyn and I catch each other's eye and try not to laugh.

Afterwards, as we walk back to collect our babies, we clutch our stomachs in fits of giggles. It feels good to laugh.

Later that night, after Henry has fallen asleep, I call Robb to tell him about the yoga.

'What's that noise?' I ask him.

'I'm pulling the roof apart. Ev's been here helping. We're putting a tarpaulin over it.'

It's a temporary solution, he tells me, until the insurers can come and assess the damage from the storm. When I hang up, Robb texts me photos of the mess on the floor and the hole where the sky streams through. It's the first time I'm grateful not to be home.

One of the women on the ward, Kylie, has a baby who is just six weeks old. She isn't allowed to leave the hospital grounds alone, but it's not until she comes with me to Burwood Westfield one afternoon that I learn why – or at least one of the reasons.

'See that bottle shop there,' Kylie says, as we push our prams out of Woolworths. 'Right now, I have this image of just smashing one of the bottles over the top of Patrick's head.'

I look at her with a well-practised poker face, careful not to betray my horror. I am, I think, less shocked by the content than the casual ease with which she shares this thought.

'It comes out of nowhere,' Kylie continues, her voice quieter as we walk down the rows of clothes shops. 'I'd never do it, though. It's horrifying. I don't understand why it happens.'

Months later, after we've both been discharged, I'll hear from Kylie via text message. Someone has reported her to DoCS and she's been asked to attend a meeting with caseworkers.

I send her a link to an article about what to expect at the meeting and remind her that she's doing all the right things. I can't help but wonder, though: was it her honesty? Did the hospital or her GP or her maternal and child health nurse, like me, blanch at her frank admission that she wanted to harm her baby?

How many children are removed from mothers like Kylie because we simply don't understand these thoughts and why they happen? How many mothers are punished by child protection for their honesty, for 'reaching out'?

We know from the research that almost all mums experience intrusive thoughts of accidentally harming their babies, while as many as half report unwanted, intrusive thoughts of harming their baby on purpose. That statistic bears repeating – as many as half. And yet it's only recently that we're beginning to understand the link between having these thoughts and the risk of *acting* on them. A 2022 study published in *The Journal of Clinical Psychiatry* found no evidence that having unwanted intrusive thoughts of intentionally harming a baby is associated with an increased risk of harm to the infant. While for most women the thoughts disappear on their own, researchers estimate about 9 per cent are at risk of developing postnatal obsessive-compulsive disorder (OCD) in the first six months after birth. This, too, can be treated but, although it's more common than previously thought, it is also often mismanaged or misdiagnosed (sometimes as postnatal psychosis).

I find myself thinking about Kylie sometimes, wondering what happened to her and how she is. I never heard from her again after that last message about DoCS, and with the possibility that a colleague might have been involved with her case, I didn't feel I could follow up too closely. But I do think of her bravery and how open she was about what was happening inside her head. Can you see, though? Are you starting to understand why I wasn't?

༄

'I can't *believe* you're getting out of art therapy,' I tell Carolyn, as we drop our babies off at the nursery.

'I'd rather colour in than see my psychiatrist,' she says. 'Want to swap?'

'Honestly, yes.'

The young woman running the art therapy class is gentle and patient. 'The room is yours,' she tells us as we walk in. 'There are paints, pencils, clay. Help yourself.'

Fiona picks out a colouring book and a box of pencils and starts shading.

'I find this more anxiety-inducing than helpful,' I say with a nervous laugh, taking a seat around the long table. 'It just reminds me how hopeless I am at drawing.'

What's the evidence base for this rubbish? I think.

'You don't have to be good at art,' the therapist says. (I suspect I'm not the first art sceptic/intellectual arsehole to enter her studio.) 'Just do what feels comfortable.'

Nothing feels comfortable.

As I write this scene, I can see myself there in that room. It's a small group of us, just mums from the mother and baby unit, and the artist is so kind and I want to reach out from here in the future and tell that belligerent twenty-something to pick up a bloody pencil or a paintbrush and stop being such a snob. 'Do some bloody art, Beeston,' I want to say. 'Stop thinking that everything is black and white. None of this is an exact science. None of it. And part of what will save you is art.'

But I don't pick up a pencil. Instead, always more comfortable with words, I cut words and phrases from glossy magazines and arrange them in a collage on a piece of cardboard.

Baby blues / It's a girl / Help / Back to work / Recover / mama /crazy / 27.9 is the average age of new mums / OK / Rebuild / get out and walk / emotional / boy meets girl / tired / struggling / magic moments / you can be a confident mum / now what / yummy mummies / sociologists wouldn't deny that the desire for a child is very strong / SOS / Girl Interrupted / deep breaths / CRY / going up going down / sobs / do you have a wife with postnatal depression?

I cut and paste and cut and paste; the hour disappears. And the relief of silence, a break from the telling and retelling of my story, is immense.

Later that evening, I take Henry for a walk to the newsagent and buy copies of three glossy magazines – the trashier the better. When we get back, I spread my 'art' on the bed and get to work. Soon, the cardboard is completely covered – word over word over word.

From my room to hers, I text Carolyn a photo of my finished

masterpiece. 'What do you reckon?' I say.

'HAHAHA,' she replies. 'Won't you look at that.'

The next morning, as I'm dressing, Henry escapes down the hallway with his baby walker – a nudie run on wheels. The nurses shriek with laughter as he reaches their station at the end of the corridor and I feel my heart burst with pride for my beautiful, cheeky boy, The Streaker. It's a new feeling and I'm giddy with it.

∽

'I'm going to write about this one day,' I tell the group at therapy towards the end of my stay. 'No one warned me about any of this.'

'I think that's a wonderful idea,' the social worker says.

Carolyn laughs. 'I'd read it.'

'I would too,' says Fiona.

When I *did* start to write about this time, I often reflected on whether I wanted to read my patient records. Would it be helpful to read the doctors' notes or would it be too painful, too confront-ing? Would my memories match up with their records?

But when I call the hospital's records department to see if I can have a copy of the mother/infant filming, the woman tells me that as my admission was more than seven years ago, all my files have been destroyed.

'Seriously?' I say. 'They're all gone?'

'Yes,' she says. 'By law we don't have to keep them for more than seven years.'

'Yeah, right. There you go.'

'There's a discharge summary here,' she says. 'Scanned to your file. I'll send you that.'

When I hang up, I'm disappointed at first, then surprised by the relief that follows. If the records had been there, I'd have felt that not accessing them would somehow be leaving part of my story out. But the decision has been taken out of my hands.

While I know it would have been strange to read notes made about me while I was so unwell, there's a sense of curiosity there too – what did they see? What did they miss? What was the narrative they strung together from the pieces I gave them – and the pieces I didn't?

⟿

Henry and I are discharged on Robb's birthday, three weeks after we were admitted. It's shorter than most stays (the average is around four weeks) but I am ready to go. I circle responses I know will add up to a lower score. The same day, Robb's sister Jacqui goes into labour with her second baby. Our new nephew, Arthur, is born later that afternoon in Brisbane. Robbs sends me a photo as I'm packing up our belongings. The baby looks just like his dad.

'You're off?' says one of the cleaners, as I'm zipping my suitcase.

'Yeah, home today.'

'That's good,' she says. 'You don't need to be in here anymore. You're doing so well.'

How easy it is to perform, I think. *How easy it is to dance when you know the steps.*

Robb arrives after work to bring us home. I hug Carolyn goodbye and tell her she won't be far behind me. She's planning to leave early next week and, as it happens, lives near my parents.

'Text me,' I say.

'I will,' Carolyn says.

When I stop by Fiona's room to say goodbye, her eyes fill with tears. She is getting better, but slower than she'd like. Her shoulders are slumped in an oversized black shirt.

'Please don't cry, or I'll start crying,' I say, covering my face.

'I'll try,' she says.

I hand her a card I've written and give her a hug.

'Hang on,' Fiona says, ripping a page out of a notebook. 'I'll give you my email address.' She writes it on the paper and folds it.

Later, I see that along with the email address she's written the words: 'Dear Henry, you are so lucky to have Ariane as your mum.'

How did she know it was exactly what I needed to read?

You're supposed to get better after you leave hospital. That's how the mental illness narrative goes. You take your new meds and your mindfulness and your fresh CBT strategies and your artwork that looks like a ransom note and your 'bad day plan' and your stress bucket diagram and you get better at 'accepting help' and busting those motherhood myths and maybe tentatively return to work and friendships and life.

If this were a novel, that's how I'd write it.

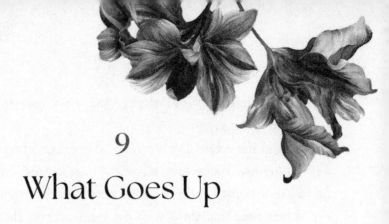

9

What Goes Up

'It's a joy to be hidden and a disaster not to be found.'

D.W. WINNICOTT

It's harder to adjust to life back at home than I thought it would be. Being in hospital was a reprieve from the world – being home is a reminder that I am still not quite part of it. The rain has stopped but the house still feels dark and damp.

I make an appointment to see Dr Wilson, running, bounding down the corridor with a huge grin. Henry is in daycare; I am free, and I am buzzing.

'I'm back!'

'You look well,' he says.

'Never better. Did you miss me?'

In years to come, as I go over my past with a highlighter trying to understand, this stands out as strange. Was I hypomanic? Did he not notice? What goes up …

⟡

As part of my discharge plan, the hospital has referred me to a local psychiatrist, a man who specialises in CBT. But when Dr Wilson phones to check his availability, they recommend a different doctor, a woman with expertise in perinatal mental health. She is also trained in CBT but she uses psychodynamic therapy as well.

'I think Dr Q will be a better fit,' the receptionist tells him. 'And she has availability. Can Ariane come in next week?'

I am sceptical, to say the least. During my training and particularly at DoCS, CBT was considered 'gold standard.' Psychodynamic therapy, with its close ties to Freud and psychoanalysis, is as foreign to me as the inkblots gathering dust in my cupboard at work. But I want to get back to work. I'm certain it will help me get better. So I say yes.

Dr Q's office is in the inner city, a train ride away. I put on a bright purple jumper, wash and blow-dry my hair and wear pink lipstick for our first session. Dr Q will later dispute this account: 'No, you wore a red jumper,' she says, 'skinny jeans and ballet flats.' We will agree to disagree.

Henry has just started at a local day care in preparation for my return to work and the newfound freedom – the unanchored space and time – is less thrilling than disorienting. I have too much time to think.

Dr Q's office is at the top of a rickety wooden staircase and when she calls my name, I follow her up and sit in a large leather chair. She is small, even shorter than me, with dark hair and beautiful skin. Behind her desk are shelves covered in books.

My story, again. A new audience, a new performance. A new agenda.

I tell Dr Q that the medication they prescribed me in hospital, mirtazapine, makes me drowsy. I can hardly function, let alone parent. Taking it at night doesn't make any difference. I don't hear Henry when he wakes and I can't get up in the morning.

'Alright, then,' Dr Q says, reading through my notes and

discharge summary. 'Let's take you off it completely and see how you go. There are other options we can try if we need to.'

'Okay,' I say. 'And I'd also like to go back to work soon. I think it would be good for me. I think it would help.'

We agree that I'll plan to go back to DoCS two days a week in about a month's time, with no clinical work initially, which the hospital psychiatrists had suggested, too.

'If you were a florist, I wouldn't be worried,' Dr Q explains. 'But you're going back to a very stressful job. I know you're keen, and I do understand why, but we'll need to take it slowly. Okay?'

I nod. I've heard it all before.

～

The first time I read the word 'psychotic' to describe my postpartum experience is in the letter Dr Q writes to Dr Wilson about two months after our first appointment. By then, I'd seen her four or five times, making my way to her office by train – clean clothes, bright lipstick.

> In summary, Ariane has suffered from a severe psychotic depression in the postnatal period. She has had significant agitation, anxiety and panic exacerbated by contemporaneous psychological stressors in this postnatal period.

Dr Q lets me read the letter in her office before she sends it. 'I like to be transparent,' she says. It's an approach I'll come to respect and admire – there are no secrets and I'm never concerned about what she might be recording in my file.

I feel relieved. There's a reason for how terrible I've felt, for how confusing and scary and painful and gutting these past ten months have been. There's a word for it – and I have always been comforted by words.

I read on.

Recovery also sadly brings with it the realisation of the gravity of her illness, the sense of a lack of agency as well as the need to tolerate potential unknowns. Ariane has expressed her poignant awareness of the loss of her first twelve months even while she appreciates her progressing recovery.

Given the side effects, I recommended that we should withdraw her antidepressant and we can carefully watch over her recovery together ... At this stage, Ariane would prefer not to be on any medication at all, let alone an antipsychotic.

She would like to return to work part-time. While her work environment appears supportive, the work itself can be vicariously traumatising, as I'm sure you are aware. However, I am confident Ariane will be able to negotiate this and continue to cautiously remain engaged with both of us to ensure that relapse is prevented or swiftly addressed.

Years later, Dr Q will tell me she was worried about how I'd react to the letter.

'But how did you *know*?' I ask her. 'I didn't tell you anything. I didn't tell you about the delusions or the hallucinations or how bad I was feeling.'

'Clinical experience,' she says. By then I've been seeing her for almost half a decade and there's humour and tenderness and safety between us. 'It was about looking at the gestalt of you. To see what was missing. Just little things. The way you spoke. Walked. There was a lot in what you didn't say, too. It made me wonder, *Hmmm, what's really going on here?*'

I thought I had hidden my madness so well. I'm glad I didn't hide it well enough.

It is a disaster not to be found.

∽

Unlike postnatal depression, which occurs in one in seven new mothers, postpartum psychosis (or puerperal psychosis) is rare – it affects around one to two in every 1000 mums. That's around 600 women in Australia each year. But for those affected, it can be debilitating and life-threatening. Postpartum psychosis is considered a psychiatric emergency. Women experience a loss of contact with reality, which can place both themselves and their babies at risk of harm. The suicide and infanticide rates associated with the illness sit at approximately 5 per cent and 4 per cent respectively.

Symptoms usually appear in the first few days or weeks after a baby is born. Unlike the antenatal period, where women are seen regularly, this often coincides with being discharged from hospital, partners returning to work and more limited engagement with health professionals. The phrase 'kaleidoscope' appears in the literature because symptoms can change rapidly. They can include high or low mood, visual, auditory or olfactory hallucinations as well as delusions (false beliefs), often but not always about the baby.

We don't know exactly what causes postpartum psychosis. Women with bipolar disorder are more at risk of developing the condition and for some women it's the first presentation of the illness. You're more likely to experience postpartum psychosis as a first-time mother, and in subsequent pregnancies if you've experienced it once before. Hormonal, immunological factors and genetic factors may also play a role, and lack of sleep is considered a potential trigger. Interestingly, adverse or stressful life events, personality and temperament do not appear to be associated with the illness.

For many women with postpartum psychosis (about 40 per cent) it occurs out of the blue. And for many families, it's the first time they've had to navigate the mental health system.

ᔧ

> 'Blackness as black as black / Black like a miner's cave / Without a light burning blue / Searching in the dark for something; / a memory, something tactile, something tangible / something to touch but finding nothing.'
>
> EMILY, FEBRUARY 2022

Emily is a little over a week postpartum and she hasn't slept for more than a few hours. Her husband, a police officer, calls an ambulance to their home in Sydney.

At first, doctors believe she is suffering from postpartum stress disorder after a traumatic 22-hour birth. She recalls being wheeled into theatre ten days earlier, a surgeon telling her the order of events: vacuum, forceps, episiotomy, emergency caesarean – and finally the possibility of a hysterectomy to save her life. It was four o'clock in the morning. Emily remembers a final numb push – her son, with her father's blue eyes, placed on her chest. In theatre, she is stitched up, sent back to her room. Visitors come and go, bring champagne and hospital flowers.

The first night, her baby, a healthy 4.2-kilogram boy, feeds and cries and sleeps. Emily, however, will not sleep for days. And it's here, she tells me, that her memories are not to be trusted.

'Normal vaginal birth,' a midwife writes on Emily's discharge notes.

'Normal?' Emily asks.

Nothing, Emily thinks, *seems normal.*

An obstetrician agrees she can remain in hospital for a few more days. Emily is seen by a psychiatric consultant, who diagnoses her with bipolar disorder and prescribes her lithium. But Emily is breastfeeding and doesn't want to stop. *Battery acid*, she thinks. Emily calls MotherSafe, the NSW counselling line for women and healthcare providers concerned about exposure to drugs during pregnancy and nursing. They tell her that if she takes lithium, she must stop breastfeeding. She ignores it – and the new diagnosis.

She wants to breastfeed, and she will.

While still in hospital, Emily texts her husband: 'I want you to read but don't use it as evidence with any medical staff don't worry but please could you share my feelings with a sensible and responsible adult. I'm trusting you with my life here and Oscar's. I get it. I also get that I wrote an essay yesterday. I'm an art and English teacher!!!'

Discharged from the ward and back at home, Emily gives her grandmother a history lesson, rambling about Hitler, Skinner, Orwell and the psychologist Stanley Milgram, who devised the electric-shock experiment to test obedience to authority. She organises a book club, launches a photography business. She visits her GP twice, tells him she's not depressed, says she feels like the Hulk.

By now, it's been ten days since she's slept properly. On the night the ambulance arrives at their home, Emily had become 'violent'. She is scheduled (admitted to hospital as an involuntary patient) under the NSW *Mental Health Act*.

This will last three-and-a-half months. ECT will be mandated.

She sends a text to her dad: 'F**k she left. We're going to die. Dad you're good. Buy gold! We're in for World War Three! Show the doctor. See you soon. Kill me before I ruin the book. A war is coming. I am going to be Shakespeare. Dad, you picked the right book. Shut up. I'll kill her but I'll never crack. I'll kill myself and I can see fuck get Ben. Get everyone I hate and love. Listen. Holy shit, you're right. Let us protect. I'm not ready To die. Kill me. I'm not ready. Time.'

She texts her friends: 'It's time. You know where to find me next week. I can see Plath. SOS.'

In Sutherland Hospital on the psychiatric ward, Emily wanders the halls trying to decode the numbers on the doors. They'll unlock the mystery of the nightmare she has found herself in. They're also the winning lottery numbers. She tells her husband to buy a lottery ticket.

She tries to feed the chickens in her room with her hospital food.

'There aren't any chickens,' her husband says.

'Yes, there are,' Emily argues. 'And you're the horse. You're Boxer, from *Animal Farm*.'

She is forced into a straitjacket. She kicks a nurse in the groin. She screams all the profanities she's ever known.

She doesn't remember any of this.

What Emily *does* remember is waking up after ECT, holding the hand of an old friend and asking if she'd been in a car accident. 'No,' her friend tells her. 'You had postpartum psychosis. You had a baby.'

'What baby?' Emily asks.

On day release from hospital, Emily buys a copy of George Orwell's *Animal Farm*, fills it with her own annotations. She sits in hospital, poring over each line, trying to decipher the mystery. Each sentence has significance.

She hasn't touched Orwell since.

I first meet Emily in the Australian and New Zealand Facebook group Beyond Postnatal Psychosis – which is now more than 200 women strong – and then on Zoom during the winter school holidays. She is warm and funny and open. We share a love of literature and swap recommendations for books and poetry.

'The Plath reference gave me a chuckle,' I say. 'I mean, it's not funny, obviously, but my psychiatrist told me to stop reading Plath. She said it was unnecessarily "amplifying".'

'I can't *stop* reading it,' Emily says with a grin. 'The Plath/Hughes comparison text is on the Year 11–12 curriculum, so I'm teaching it.'

Although it's school holidays, Emily is in her office, catching up on work before term three begins. The swiftness of her recovery from such profound illness has surprised everyone – her doctors, her husband and even herself. Emily was back in a classroom just two months after being discharged from hospital. She began with one day a week, gradually building up to what is now a full-time teaching load of Visual Arts, including HSC students.

'I wanted to go back to work because I thought at least I knew how to do that,' Emily says. 'I know how to teach. I know I can teach Year 7 and 8 Art.'

Emily has since attained the rank of lieutenant in the Australian Defence Force. She's also been promoted to the position of training company commander.

'When I applied for the role, the Defence Force asked if I had any current medical conditions,' she says. 'I said no because I didn't have psychosis any longer. But the next question was do you take any medication? At the time I was still taking lithium daily. But the unit commander advocated for me, and I completed the required training to become a qualified lieutenant in the Second Brigade.' She laughs. 'On my health card it says, "Trigger: childbirth".'

Still, there are moments now when she wonders, *Is this a lucid dream or is it psychosis again?* On a recent cadet camp, Emily was overheating in a sleeping bag. 'I dreamt I was being pinned down on a lino floor and just really out of it,' she says. 'The way I analyse it is that I was in a psych ward, and I was being pinned down and medicated. But I couldn't throw the doona off, so I woke up screaming. Another officer was unzipping his tent to come and save me from myself and I said, "It's okay, just a nightmare." My heart was racing and pounding. So, you recover,' she says, 'but you can still have nightmares occasionally and they can happen when you're on camp.'

Aside from the dreams, Emily says her memory is fragmented and she has severe memory loss. 'Doctors said that if after six months things didn't come back, they wouldn't. And they haven't.' Her husband is reluctant to fill in the gaps, including what happened the night he called an ambulance. 'He doesn't like to talk about it for my own safety. He says, "You don't want to know." But you kind of do want to know.'

While being treated in hospital, Emily underwent a total of twenty-four sessions of ECT. 'In Prince of Wales,' she says, 'they had an ECT machine where they attach the electrodes to different areas of the brain, to where your memories are.' At St John of God, she underwent a final session of ECT, this time voluntarily. 'I thought, *Stop fighting the system, start being part of it.*' It was a stark change from the months she spent sectioned under the *Mental Health Act*. 'Initially, I hated most medical staff because I was paranoid and thought they were out to get me, but they weren't. I can now say I've met and been supported by some of the most compassionate people in the world.'

She knows she's lucky to be alive. 'If I hadn't received treatment, I probably would have ended my life, not because I was depressed but because I genuinely believed I was a type of martyr against a corrupt government. I remember trying to find the cyanide tooth capsule with my tongue discreetly. It wasn't there. Surprise. I'm not and never was an imprisoned Cold War spy agent.'

Despite it all, Emily wants to have more children – even though the risk of another episode of postpartum psychosis is high. 'I recently cuddled my cousin's six-month-old baby,' she says. 'Usually, I avoid holding tiny babies because I don't feel I learnt how to do it correctly. He was so small and fell asleep in my arms. It was such a beautiful cuddle. I realised that I wanted this feeling again with my baby – I don't think I had that same feeling with my son at six months.'

Writing stories and poems is helping Emily make sense of what she's been through – a process she describes as more akin to acceptance than post-traumatic growth (where some people experience growth or positive changes after trauma). She is also revisiting the notes she took while hospitalised. 'You can see the deterioration. It was like Brett Whiteley when he was using heroin and would write on the walls. My diary became a visual representation of my mind.'

Emily laughs. 'Halfway through I wrote: "It's hard being God."'

⏳

Emily's copy of *Animal Farm* is covered in black scribbles and orange texta. Not long after we speak for the first time, she sends me a scanned copy over email with some pages from the journals she kept while in hospital.

'Don't read them if you're not feeling well enough,' she warns me. 'They are funny but they are also very triggering!'

We postpartum sisters look after one another. I wait until after work to open them.

> *Strange dream*
> *Before I die*
> *Are rats comrades?*
> *The milk had disappeared.*

In one of Emily's journals, I find the words: 'It is hard to ask for help. Winnicott – psychologist – "be good enough".'

✍

A few weeks later we meet for a drink at a pub in Summer Hill. It's not long after I've phoned the hospital, seeking my records from my MBU stay. 'I was wondering if they had the video,' I say. 'You know, when they do the filming.'

'Oh right,' Emily snickers. 'I just said no to that.'

'Seriously?'

'Yep. I did everything else,' she says. 'But I didn't want to do that.'

'Ha,' I say. 'It didn't even occur to me that I could say no.'

In some ways, Emily says, she met the criteria of risk factors. 'They say sleep deprivation and the hormonal shift of your milk coming in can make you more vulnerable. And yes, I had a long labour and a traumatic birth. Sexual assault is also another tipping point.'

But none of her relatives have bipolar disorder or schizophrenia. Even now, there's only a pending dash against bipolar disorder – Emily's psychiatrist is waiting to see if she has another episode over the next twelve months before diagnosing her with the condition. Even though she tried to electrocute herself – 'not to die but to end Big Brother's regime' – Emily says she was never depressed after having her baby. 'I'm a unique entity.' She laughs. 'I wasn't textbook postpartum psychosis.'

What is textbook, though? I wonder. For the more I learn and the more I listen, the more I realise just how wide and varied our experiences are.

⌇

What happens when the mental illness you've experienced isn't actually in the textbook at all? That's the case for postpartum psychosis, which doesn't appear in the psychiatrists' 'bible', the DSM. 'Neither ICD [International Classification of Diseases] nor the DSM recognises postpartum psychosis as a distinct disorder,' notes *The Lancet* in a 2021 editorial. Instead, cases are classified as either general mania or psychotic depression, with an onset in the perinatal period.

'Psychotic depression' – the words I first saw written down in that letter from Dr Q.

Even I was confused about what I'd experienced. As I started to recover and research my own psychotic break, the different terminology left my head spinning.

'What's the difference between what I had – psychotic depression postpartum – and postnatal psychosis?' I once asked Dr Q during a session.

'They're the same thing,' Dr Q said.

'Oh,' I remember saying. 'Right.'

That postpartum psychosis isn't listed in the DSM or the ICD is something experts are increasingly identifying as an issue. Curiously, it used to be there. In fact, postpartum psychosis was listed in the first DSM, in 1952, as Involutional Psychotic Reaction: 'Some cases are characterized chiefly by depression and others chiefly by paranoid ideas.' In the DSM-II in 1968, it was listed as Psychosis with Childbirth. It was removed in 1980, however, disappearing from the DSM-III and the DSM-IIIR. Why? That is less clear, although the term postpartum wasn't completely removed until 1994.

I come across a 2020 petition started by Wendy Davis, the executive director of Postpartum Support International, requesting that the American Psychiatric Association recognise postpartum psychosis in their next edition of the DSM. At the time the petition had garnered almost 50,000 signatures. And the reasons for signing make compelling reading.

> I am a two-time 'Maternal Psychosis' survivor, and it was much worse than getting a Breast Cancer diagnosis. At least the term cancer wasn't deleted from medical literature for twenty (20) years like 'postpartum' was. If it had been, I'd not be here, and it nearly stands true for postpartum psychosis.

> Our daughter took her own life suffering postpartum psychosis one week after delivering her son. She was thirty-one and her first child. It happened so fast, we had no time or knowledge to seek help or an appropriate place to take her for help.

> Were this a male disorder, it would already be covered.

But the petition didn't work – postpartum psychosis wasn't included in the DSM-V. In its current format, the diagnostic information relevant to psychosis notes that perinatal-onset mood episodes can present with or without psychotic symptoms.

> Infanticide is most often associated with postpartum psychotic episodes that are characterized by command hallucinations to kill the infant or delusions that the infant is possessed, but psychotic symptoms can also occur in severe postpartum mood episodes without such specific delusions or hallucinations.

Does diagnosis really matter? It's a question I consider regularly, as do many who work in psychology or psychiatry, and many of us who've been given labels or played DSM bingo with our own brains. I'm not the only one who was confused by my diagnosis – in many online forums relating to postpartum psychosis, women from around the world are often left trying to decipher discharge notes: puerperal psychosis, mania or bipolar disorder triggered by childbirth, schizoaffective disorder with onset after delivery, depression with psychotic features.

The answer is complex – and depends on who you ask. 'The DSM is American, of course and it's a very political document,' Professor Anne Buist tells me, adding that it has many flaws. 'It is used in court,' although, she admits, less so here in Australia. 'I still have to have diagnostic criteria, but you can say you're using the English guidelines rather than the American. They're not quite so bound to it here.'

I listen to a webinar about postpartum psychosis with Dr Lee Cohen of Massachusetts General Hospital, who notes that while diagnostic issues exist, what's important is patient care. 'You can go to meetings where there are these hot debates about diagnostically what postpartum psychosis is and is not,' he says. 'But I think sometimes we miss perhaps one of the most critical pieces, which at the end of the day is that women get effective treatment and we pull together resources.'

That's certainly not up for debate.

In my own work with DoCS, I hadn't come across the term postpartum psychosis (only postnatal depression). More broadly, I had heard of postnatal depression through severe high-profile examples such as Andrea Yates (who I'll talk about in more detail in a later chapter). So I'm surprised when a friend who recently undertook child protection caseworker training tells me postpartum psychosis is now included as a case study in one of their modules. And while I'm curious about the decision to profile something far less prevalent than other perinatal mental health conditions, this recognition is surely a positive step.

Because postpartum psychosis is rare (although this too is contested in PP circles, with some suggesting that calling it 'rare' reinforces the idea that 'it won't happen to me'), it's difficult to both fund and complete research and much of what has been done is from overseas. But I do find a local paper written in 2021 by Diana Jefferies of Western Sydney University called 'The River of Postnatal Psychosis'. Jefferies and her colleagues interviewed ten women from around the country about their experience of the illness. All the women had profound sleep difficulties, with some only sleeping for short periods and others not sleeping at all. They all said they noticed a change in their personalities, such as increased anxiety or behaviours that were out of character. And they all described hallucinations and/or delusions, with some saying they did not feel able to tell anyone about it due to stigma. As one woman described:

> I had this thought that Pseudoephedrine was a wonder drug, and if I gave it to [my child] that her verbal development would

just take off. I'm thankful that I didn't act on that, because I'm sure that I could have harmed her, and other thoughts started becoming on the spiritual side, that the devil was everywhere and he was going to harm my children and I needed to protect them, and so at one point when [my partner] left me at home with [my baby], I think he was taking his sister home, I thought I need to protect her and actually she needs my blood on her to protect her.

A common theme was that even when the women asked for help and shared some of their symptoms, they were often minimised or put down to being a normal part of adjusting to motherhood. And when they finally received treatment, recovery was often slow. One line stands out for me: 'The women had to learn to survive.'

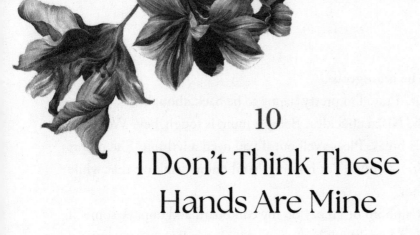

10
I Don't Think These Hands Are Mine

*'Illness exposes ... You're down to the floor of who you
are in the presence of illness.'*

DR RITA CHARON

I return to my job as a DoCS psychologist in south-west Sydney
eight weeks after I'm discharged from hospital. I've withdrawn
from all medication, I'm still seeing Dr Q, and Henry is settled
into a local childcare centre. I am nervous but excited – being
back at work will be good for me. It will help me remember who
I was before I got sick.

When I try on my work wardrobe the week before, all my
clothes are too big. I am smaller than I was before I had Henry –
still scrawny from having breastfed and months of no appetite
that's only just creeping back.

'Ariane!' Nisha, our office manager, greets me with a smile.
'How are you? How's Henry?'

'Good!' I say, showing her photos of him on my phone. Nobody
but my team leader knows where I've been and I'm grateful for
the lack of questions. As far as anyone knows, I've simply been on
maternity leave.

'Oh, he is gorgeous.'

'He is,' I say. 'I'm pretty happy to be back, though.'

'Yeah,' Nisha chuckles. 'Being a mum is tough, hey? Work can feel like a break. Please yell out if you need anything.' She points at the cup of coffee I'm holding. 'And enjoy drinking that while it's still hot.'

I put a photo of Henry on my corkboard and unpack some of the books I bought while on maternity leave. Because everything in the department moves so slowly, not much has changed in the last year. There are over one thousand emails in my inbox. By the end of the day, I have several case consults booked in and a file to review for a senior colleague who is swamped with work. He's been allocated to assess a sibling group of four and I take one of the siblings off his plate.

File reviews are familiar – a little like putting together an affidavit for the court. Often, by the time a child comes to the attention of a DoCS psychologist there are at least three or four files of information. There are the initial helpline reports, some-times just the one critical incident, sometimes a series of escalating events. There's court paperwork – affidavits, long-term care plans and final court orders. There are school reports and assessments by various clinicians – medication reviews from psychiatrists, IQ tests from school counsellors. There are behaviour management plans and contact reports from family. It's methodical, quiet work and I'm grateful for it.

But I am not the same clinician I was before I went on mater-nity leave. Perhaps this seems an obvious statement; how could I be? And yet the change in how I see everything – in the con-sults, the file reviews, the documents I'm reading – is pervasive.

Working on a transition plan for a baby who is to be moved into a short-term placement makes me physically ache. The baby is eight months old, a critical period, and has been in the same placement since he was removed at birth. It was only meant to be temporary, however, and the foster carers can no longer care for him. There are still months of court ahead before final orders are made and the child is either restored to his parents or placed with a long-term carer.

I think of Henry at the same age.

Coming back as a mother feels different.

Coming back as a mother is fucking devastating.

∽

After a consult with a child protection caseworker I log onto the KIDS system, where digital case files live. It's where we record notes on phone calls and home visits. As I'm scrolling, I see a case note about the children's mother – she spent time as an inpatient at the same hospital as me, a few years before my own admission. When I read on, I discover that her kids are no longer in her care.

She was just like me, I think, as I scan the notes and close the file. It's too raw, too close, too deep.

You are a fraud.

You don't belong here.

Imagine thinking a broken mother can do this job.

∽

Two weeks later, I'm on my way home from work, pushing Henry in the pram, when he turns into a dragon, angry and red. It's just a flash, but it's there – and then it's gone. I pull the hood of the pram down so no one else can see him.

165

When I look down, my hands are attached to me, but they're not mine. I inspect them like a scientist might. They're at the end of my arms, their fingers bear my rings, but they're still not mine.

I keep pushing the pram and call Dr Q.

'Henry looks like a dragon.'

Her voice walks me home, past Redfern Station and onto our street. I fumble in my bag for my keys. Robb is away and my stomach drops when I can't find them. But they're there in the nappy bag, stashed under the pram.

Inside, I set Henry up in his highchair with dinner and switch on ABC Kids. I lie on the ground, still dressed in my work clothes. Tears spill from my eyes. I can't seem to move. It's almost six weeks to the day since I stopped taking any medication. Going without medication hasn't worked. I have failed at that too.

I call Robb in LA – or is it Singapore? It goes through to voicemail.

'I don't feel so good,' I tell him when he calls later. 'It feels like it's all coming back.'

'Have you called Dr Q?'

'Yes, I'm seeing her tomorrow.'

'Can you call your parents?'

'Okay.'

'Please call them, Arns. It stresses me out being so far away.'

'I will.'

⟳

'We'll have to put you on something else, dear,' Dr Q says. 'And we have to protect your sleep.'

I have made it into her office the next day, after getting Henry to day care. I have stopped trying to pretend. My hair is unwashed. I don't wear lipstick. I do not smile. I wear neither purple nor red.

After just three weeks back, I am already signed off from work – away on sick leave that I do not have. This failure seems particularly shameful, perhaps because it is visible – so clearly on display. Dr Q gives me a certificate for a month off, which I fax through to my boss. I begin a course of Lexapro (another SSRI), as well as Seroquel, an antipsychotic. The first time I take it, it is so strong I sleep until two p.m. When I wake, I am groggy and disoriented.

I see Dr Q twice a week and Dr Wilson once a week. I am a full-time patient. I have failed at recovery, too.

～

Nathan moves into the vacant terrace house next door when Henry is about eleven months old. He is quiet, with small dark eyes, and keeps to himself initially. Because I am home now, again, often with nowhere to be, I get to know him slowly, in snatches. Nathan tells me he's trying to lose weight and quit smoking. He goes for long walks around the back streets of Redfern.

When spring arrives and the weather gets warmer, I sit outside on the front porch, letting Henry push his walker up and down. Sometimes Nathan joins me, sitting on his front step with a beer.

'Down 30 kilos,' he tells me one afternoon, with a grin. 'Doc's pleased.'

'You look really well,' I tell him.

'I feel much better,' he says. 'Much better. How are you?'

'Good, thanks,' I say.

'Little fella keeping you busy?'

'Always.'

〜

'I don't feel safe with these,' I tell Dr Wilson, handing him the box of Valium he prescribed to help with my anxiety and increasing panic attacks. These attacks come from nowhere and everywhere and leave me gasping for breath, often curled in the fetal position or ensconced in Robb's arms. My fingers tingle and my legs forget how to work. 'I don't want them in my house.' Dr Wilson cuts off a strip of five tablets and hands them to me, then puts the rest of the packet in his drawer. 'We're going to get you through this, Ariane,' he tells me. 'We're going to get you better.'

My memory of this time is blurry and fragmented. Colourless. I see death everywhere: in the medication I take each night, on the escalators at the shopping centres. I catch the train to visit Dr Q and see myself falling onto the tracks.

I am terrified of the sun, of going outside. I am obsessed with UV rays, paranoid that they will harm me and Henry. I believe they are sentient beings out to get us – but only us. We do not leave the house until my phone says the UV index is less than three. If the sun is too hot on my skin, I panic and rush us back home. I pull the curtains shut to block out the light.

'Is he sunburnt?' I text Robb photographs of Henry when we're safe inside the house, one after the other. 'Can you see it? He's burnt, isn't he? It's my fault.'

'He looks fine to me, Arns,' Robb says. Ever patient, ever kind. 'I'm on my way home.'

We try to laugh – it's like the nappy rash, only this time my brain is focused on the sun. But it is exhausting. We are exhausted. I am exhausting.

Even now, the smell of sunscreen makes me anxious.

Years later, I'll watch the TV series *Better Call Saul*. One of its main characters, Chuck, has an electromagnetic hypersensitivity. In one scene, Chuck ventures outside covered in a foil blanket. Everything is heightened – the sounds of the street, the lights – and he appears in physical pain.

'Holy shit,' I tell Robb. 'That's what it felt like when I went out into the sun. That's exactly what it felt like. Like all the UV rays were out to get us and I couldn't keep us safe.'

❦

I'm early for my appointment with Dr Q, so I sit in the park across from her office. It's a warm, sunny day and the grass is dotted with office workers having lunch. I am taking my book out of my bag when I see it – the most perfect leaf. I pick it up carefully and turn it around. It is beautifully proportioned, as though someone has drawn it.

I set it down against the cover of my book and take photos of it, sending them to Robb in quick succession.

'Look at this leaf!' I say. 'Have you ever seen a more beautiful leaf?'

'It's a nice leaf,' Robb replies. 'I guess.'

'It's more than nice!' I text him. 'Look at it. It's the most perfect leaf I've ever seen. Have you ever seen anything more beautiful?'

Preoccupied with the leaf, I realise I am almost late for my appointment. I am never late. I grab my bag and run across the road.

'Dr Q!' I exclaim when she lets me into the office. 'Look at this! Have you ever seen anything more perfect?'

Dr Q raises an eyebrow and takes the leaf from me.

'You're a little elevated today.'

'Am I?'

'A little.' She hands it back and I fold it into the pages of my book.

Later that afternoon, it starts to rain on my way to collect Henry from day care. I log onto Twitter.

@arianebeeston: Hello lovely rain!

@arianebeeston: Seriously put your face to the sky it's a delight!

@arianebeeston I haven't been drinking this is just a nice joyful tweet!

✍

Have I mentioned the hypomania yet? Hypomania feels like flying. It feels like light and love and happiness so intense I think I might crack from its sheer strength. I make aggressive eye contact with men in the street, holding it for three seconds too long. I could take any of them. They all want me. In the mirror, my reflection shines. I am more beautiful than I have ever been. I will write the next great novel. I dance and laugh and dance and laugh and I am funny, so very funny. My brain makes connections between words and phrases and ideas and I am creative and brilliant and I dance and dance and dance and dance.

And I crash.

✍

Lizzie has a baby, a much longed-for baby – a perfect brown-eyed boy.

The day after he is born, I plan to visit her for a few hours while Henry is in day care. I head to Kmart to buy singlets and tiny socks to take with me as a present. Just three weeks earlier I'd drunk champagne and eaten cupcakes with Lizzie's friends and family at her baby shower. It was the first time I'd been social in a long time, the first time I'd felt 'normal'.

As I'm leaving the shopping centre to catch a bus to the maternity ward, I have a panic attack. My heart starts beating too fast. My legs wobble beneath me and my eyes fill with tears.

'I am so sorry,' I text Lizzie, from a bathroom cubicle where I take refuge until the panic quietens. 'I'm having a panic attack. In the toilets. I just don't think I can get there.'

'It's okay, my love!' she texts back. 'Of course this is hard. Come visit when we're home.'

I am terrified of being around a newborn. I had no idea I was so scared.

∽

Our neighbour Nathan's nephew, Adam, moves in with him. He is in his early twenties and arrives one day with cardboard boxes and an old car. The two of them scream at each other, often late at night and into the early hours of the morning. It's clear Adam is dealing from the house – people come and go at strange times.

One day, in passing, Nathan tells Robb that Adam has been stealing his medication and selling it.

'Sorry about the noise,' Nathan says. 'I keep telling him you've got the little fella.'

Nathan never tells me his diagnosis, but I come to believe that he lives with schizophrenia. There are other times when Robb and I hear him next door yelling or screaming or crying out in what sounds like pain or terror.

Some nights he turns the vacuum on at three a.m., bashing it against the stairwell as he cleans the house. Occasionally, an ambulance arrives and takes him away. Sometimes he's gone for a few days, sometimes a few weeks.

'He's gettin' big,' Nathan always says of Henry whenever he returns. We never talk about his hospital stays. I never tell him about mine.

I am lonely and he is lonely too.

⟨ℑ⟩

I am pushing Henry in the pram back home after spending the afternoon at the park when I see a crowd standing outside the front of our house. There's a police car, several police officers and a pair of detectives in dark suits.

'He did it,' Adam says to me, when he sees us coming around the corner. 'He fucken did it.' His eyes are red and he is shuffling from one foot to the other.

'Did what?'

'They let him out of hospital and he jumped off the roof. He's dead.'

'Oh fuck.' I put my hand over my mouth.

I'm conscious then of the police, watching us both. We are surrounded.

'I'm so sorry,' I say, pushing through. 'I have to get Henry inside and give him dinner, but I'm next door if you need anything. Robb will be home soon, too. Just ask.'

'Thanks, mate.'

Three days later, I am home with Henry when two detectives – a man and a woman – ring the doorbell.

'Good afternoon,' the man says, introducing himself. He has blond hair and a blond moustache. 'We'd like to talk to you about Nathan. Ask you a couple of questions. We understand you knew him?'

'A little,' I say. 'I mean, he lived next door for a bit, and I've been on mat leave.' I'm not sure whether I'm supposed to invite them inside. The floor is covered in toys and the kitchen is a mess. 'I'm not really sure what I can tell you.'

'We'd like to get a statement from you,' the woman says. 'We are trying to understand what happened.' She's in a grey suit and isn't much older than me. 'Can you please come up to the station?'

'Now?'

'If that's okay, yes. We can do it up the road at Redfern.'

I look over at where Henry is feeding a cracker to the cat.

'Well, I have my son,' I say. 'My husband is out.'

'That's okay,' the man says. 'It won't take long.' He looks at Henry and back at me. 'Unfortunately, we can't give you a lift because we don't have a car seat. But we'll meet you up there.'

At the station, the detectives usher me through to an inter-view room upstairs. I hand the female detective my phone and tell her that Henry can watch *Peppa Pig* videos on YouTube. The male detective is a painfully slow typist. He asks me questions about Nathan, about his routine and the services who came and went in the time he lived next door. I answer them with half an eye on Henry, who has the female detective chasing him up and down the corridor. She looks exhausted and relieved when Robb arrives.

'You okay?' Robb asks me, picking up the crackers Henry has rubbed into the carpet.

'Yeah,' I say with a sigh. 'Almost done. I'll walk home.'

When I tell Dr Q about the detectives at my next appoint-ment, she is pissed off.

'Why didn't you say it wasn't a convenient time and they could come back when it was?'

'I didn't think I could.'

'We're going to work on that.'

❦

The day of Nathan's funeral is hot and humid. It's October and storm clouds roll overhead as we drive into the car park at the cemetery in Western Sydney. There are only about six or seven of us inside the chapel, including Adam and the two detectives. The female detective smiles. The male detective doesn't. I wonder what they're doing here.

We take a seat at the back, and I put my head on Robb's shoulder. I have felt leaden since waking up – my brain full of stones, my heart a ghost. Even though I didn't know Nathan very well, I cry for him.

'Suicide is a permanent solution to a temporary problem,' the funeral celebrant says. I've since heard this expression many times, but that day in the hot chapel, surrounded by people I didn't know, was the first. It didn't feel comforting or fair or helpful, and its use at a funeral for a man who'd taken his own life makes me seethe. I've never forgotten it.

I'll never forget it or Nathan.

❦

'I don't think I'm ever going to get better,' I say to Dr Q. I am slumped in her chair. The world has slowed once more. When I walk, it is through mud. The left side of me aches again. I am floating somewhere between sickness and health, around and around in the betweenness of it. I am a burden to Robb. I am ruining his life. I have ruined my career. Why would anyone want to stay with me?

'You will get better,' she says. 'This illness is an assault on the brain. It will take time.' I think about what my brain must look like – I imagine where the damage might live and what colour it might be, what shape, what scars we cannot see.

She was right, of course. I would get better. She just couldn't tell me exactly when.

'I don't understand how this happened. I don't know how I got here,' I say.

'You are trying to make sense of what doesn't make sense,' Dr Q responds. She is right about that, too.

You have to break to rebuild – and so you break: down to go up. Down to go up.

I become obsessed with death. I read *Staring at the Sun* by psychiatrist Irvin Yalom: 'Though the physicality of death destroys us, the idea of death saves us.' I read Nabokov's *Speak, Memory*: 'The cradle rocks above an abyss, and common sense tells us that our existence is but a brief crack of light between two eternities of darkness.' I look at the empty space on the steps where Nathan used to sit and wonder how he felt when he made the decision to go. When did he know?

I am ready to die, but I need to confront my fear of death. I stare at it. I am ready to die. It is ready for me.

Not yet. But soon.

∽

It's Christmas Eve. I am so low I can hardly move. My limbs are heavy again. We have travelled to Brisbane for Christmas with Robb's family and are staying in a hotel nearby. Jacqui, Nick, Bella and Arthur have been living in Robb's parents' house, so there's no room for us at the inn.

From bed, I text Dr Q: 'I don't feel good.' I am under the starchy sheets, curtains closed. Henry and Robb are in the city for some last-minute Christmas shopping, so I am alone. How to explain that my blood feels grey?

'I think we might try adding some lamotrigine when you get back,' Dr Q replies. We have talked about this medication before – it's a mood stabiliser, yet another drug to add to the cocktail I've tried. I don't want more drugs in my already sluggish system, but I am just so tired of trying to stay alive. I don't care anymore.

'Okay,' I say. 'Merry Christmas, Dr Q.'

'Merry Christmas, dear.'

A week later, I'm standing in my parents' kitchen. We're back in Sydney, exchanging Christmas presents and eating my nonna's mince pies. I can hear Henry splashing in the pool with Evan and Amy when the text message arrives. One of the babies in my mothers' group, a little one whose mother I had become particularly close to, has died over Christmas. Later, we will learn it was from a rare virus, one that attacks the brain. But we don't know that now. All we know now is that she was sick, like all kids at day care get sick, and two days later she was gone.

Robb holds me as I sob into his shirt. Mum brings me a cup of milky instant coffee and Dad hands me a box of tissues. Evan and Amy take Henry into the living room, where I hear the beginning of his favourite movie, *Cars*.

We sit at the kitchen table in silence. My beautiful aunt Glyn and uncle Greg lost two babies, both shortly after they were born. We are thinking of Henry's little friend and her parents. We are thinking of my aunt and uncle's babies and we are all still in this grief.

The next day is New Year's Eve. I take a Valium and go to bed at eight p.m.

How selfish to want to die, to want to end your life. You selfish, selfish bitch.

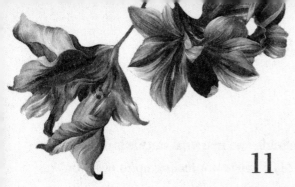

11
How Did the Baby Live?

*'Where subjects are predisposed to mental illness through
either hereditary antecedents, previous illnesses, or
through an excessive nervous susceptibility, pregnancy,
delivery and lactation can have disastrous repercussions.'*

LOUIS-VICTOR MARCÉ, *TREATISE ON INSANITY IN
PREGNANT, POSTPARTUM, AND LACTATING WOMEN* (1858)

During lockdown, instead of baking bread, I work my way through
every single episode of *Grey's Anatomy*. In one episode, a mother
drives her car with her two children off a bridge. I am in the early
stages of writing this book proposal and scribble down the following exchange between Dr Callie Torres and Dr Meredith Grey.

> Callie: Is she one of those crazy mums who tries to drown
> her kids?
> Meredith: Maybe she needed a nanny.

Actually, as they go on to discover, she had a fucking brain
tumour.

∽

This next section about infanticide and maternal suicide is difficult reading, so perhaps skip over it if you're not feeling up to it. If you do read on, I urge you to take care. I have chosen to include these topics because – while rare – cases of severe perinatal mental illness can have utterly tragic outcomes. It's also important that if we can, we don't look away. We cannot afford to keep looking away. Identifying such severe illness and treating it is crucial.

It's been over twenty years since Andrea Yates drowned her five children in Houston, Texas: seven-year-old Noah, five-year-old John, three-year-old Paul, two-year-old Luke and six-month-old Mary. An article about her case, published in *The Lancet*, notes:

> In jail, Andrea said she had considered killing the children for two years. She had not been a good mother to them, she said; they were not developing correctly. She claimed to have been marked by Satan, and that the only way to save her children from hell was to kill them. Then, when the state punished her for their deaths, Satan himself would be destroyed. Television cartoon characters told her she was a bad mother. She heard a human voice that told her to get a knife. On the walls of the jail, she saw satanic teddy bears and ducks. She said she was not mentally ill and had never been depressed because she had never cried.

Although she has been diagnosed with several different conditions – including bipolar disorder, schizophrenia and major depression – postnatal psychosis is, according to *The Lancet*, 'the most definitive'.

In her incredible book *Therapy and the Postpartum Woman*, Karen Kleiman reflects on Yates's story and the false belief that it may encourage others who are struggling to seek help. In fact, it has had the opposite effect. 'A mother who has lost touch with reality is a concept that is difficult to grasp,' writes Kleiman, who adds that it's why the attention-grabbing headlines of stories such as Yates's are so distressing. 'The bizarre nature of the symptoms and behaviours associated with psychosis is incomprehensible to those who are thinking in rational organized ways.'

In 2022, a Melbourne mother, M.A., pleaded guilty to infanticide after she lay herself and her baby on railway tracks. M.A. survived but her three-month-old baby was killed. The young mum was later diagnosed with severe postpartum depression and psycho-sis, including auditory hallucinations telling her that she was not good enough and to take her own life. She also believed there was something wrong with her baby – in this case, that the baby was suffering from shaken baby syndrome.

Under the *Crimes Act*, infanticide recognises the role that post-partum mental illness can play in such tragedies. Reading the judgement after I've learnt about the diagnostic issues around postnatal psychosis is eye-opening.

> Professor Holmes opined that at the time of the incident you were psychotic and clearly of a disturbed mind, suffering severe postpartum major depression with psychotic features consequent to the birth of your daughter three months previously. Your postpartum depression occurred on a background of compli-cated delivery and a perfectionistic self-critical personality style.
>
> [Professor Anne Buist] diagnosed you with a postpartum psychosis and explained that this is an affective psychosis, likely

a variant of bipolar disorder. She also indicated that in DSM-V terms you experienced a major depressive illness with psychotic features occurring in the postpartum period.

The judgement also noted that a diagnosis of postpartum psychosis wasn't made until after the baby's death.

It is apparent that no one understood, at that time, the extent to which your judgement and decision-making were impaired by delusional thinking and frank psychosis. The fact that your postpartum depression was overlooked is an unfortunate feature that this case has in common with certain other cases of infanticide.

'Unfortunate feature' is an understatement.

I can't help but see the similarities with my own life – the perfectionism, the 'complicated delivery', the fact that no one picked up on just how bad things were.

While writing this chapter, the outcomes of two other tragic cases are reported in the media. The first is of Sydney mother Roberta Seville (a pseudonym), who drowned her four-month-old in the bath. 'Friends and family saw her on occasion to be "not herself" and "spaced out", said Justice Button in his judgement.

Two eminent and highly experienced forensic psychiatrists firmly hold the shared opinion that, at the time, the accused suffered from perinatal major depression with psychotic features to it. I approach the latter phrase as meaning that, in more than one way, the thinking and feelings of the accused were thoroughly divorced from reality.

The second case is of a Melbourne midwife who sought help from ten different medical professionals before taking the life of her six-month-old baby, Spencer, and attempting to take her own. She was seen by three GPs, three psychologists and four emergency department staff while trying to access help during the pandemic.

'I just wonder whether in some ways, the system is not seeing the things it should see, with risks to both mother and child?' said Supreme Court judge Justice Lex Lasry.

Professor Buist is quoted in the judgement:

It is my considered view from this history and examination that Ms Nguyen's state of mind was disturbed and significantly impaired ... altered by giving birth and lactation, both triggers for her developing depressive and obsessional thinking that ultimately became psychotic ... She was predisposed to mental illness perinatally because of her genetics and personality style, but giving birth destabilised her, altering the balance of her mind such that there was a resulting psychotic illness that affected her ability to make sense of her thoughts and make decisions in a rational manner.

Coverage of the case is everywhere, unnecessarily, and desperately sad. I don't read comments on the many articles published online – they are thick with ignorance and violence. There is still so much stigma and so much misunderstanding.

In a statement provided by the midwife and her husband, published in the *Herald Sun*, the couple asked for their baby's death to be a learning experience for health care about the vulnerability of women after giving birth.

This was a tragedy that could have been avoided. She reached out for help – and many women will not do this – and the system is not equipped and it's not ready to give the kind of assistance that she needed. The assistance she received only occurred when the crisis occurred, and when the tragedy of her son's death occurred.

Families and women need more support when it comes to postnatal depression. It is a condition surrounded by shame and stigma which makes women hesitant to seek help when – as His Honour said – it is supposed to be a happy time, and they are struggling.

The family want Spencer's legacy to be one of healthcare change and reform, 'where women can feel safe to speak about their post-natal and perinatal experience and for a system to develop so that this tragedy can be avoided from the beginning of a woman's jour-ney into motherhood, all the way through to when she asks for help and when she really needs it'.

I hadn't been back at work for long, perhaps a few weeks, when Manhattan lawyer Cynthia Wachenheim jumped to her death from an eight-storey window in Harlem, with her ten-month-old baby strapped to her chest. The little boy survived, cushioned by his mother. When she died, Cynthia left a thirteen-page suicide note, writing that what she was about to do was 'evil'. 'I love him so much, but it's obviously a terrible kind of love,' she wrote.

It's a love where I can't bear knowing he is going to suffer phys-ically and mentally/emotionally for much of his life ... I wanted to be a mother so badly and I hoped to be a wonderful one, and instead I have become the worst of the worst.

Cynthia believed that her son had brain damage – and that it was her fault. In the note, she shared that her son had taken a few tumbles, including 'two shameful incidents', a fall from a play set onto the wood floor when she walked out of the room for five minutes, and off a bed. But although Cynthia consulted doctors and her family, no one could convince her that her baby was healthy and unharmed. She began to believe that he would have been better off not being born.

An article in *The New York Times* notes that Wachenheim was someone people 'didn't think they had to worry about'. Her sister Deb told the paper, 'We did try to help her, but perhaps if we had been more knowledgeable about postpartum mood disorders, including the fact that postpartum depression is just one array of such mood disorders, we could have done something differently that would have maybe saved her life.'

Years later, one of my favourite poets, Maggie Smith, will write a poem about her:

> *... the new mother strapped*
>
> *her infant to her chest, opened*
> *the eighth-floor window*
>
> *and jumped ...*
>
> *how did the baby live? Look,*
> *he smiles and totters around*
>
> *the apartment eight stories up.*

Cynthia had no history of mental illness and showed no symptoms of depression or anxiety until her son was four months old.
She was seeing a psychiatrist and had seen her son's paediatrician
multiple times. But no one knew how unwell she was. And no one
picked up that she was psychotic.

Here in Australia, the Gidget Foundation was created in the
memory of a mother, Louise, whose nickname was Gidget. She
took her own life while suffering from severe postnatal depression.
Her baby, Jasmine, was just nine months old.

'Back then I knew nothing about postnatal depression,' said her
mother, Sue Cotton, during a Gidget Foundation Australia event.

Lou had seen a new GP who diagnosed her as having mild
postnatal depression. He gave her a referral letter to Tresillian
and some medication but no counselling. He took some blood
and asked her to come back in a week. She spoke to Tresillian,
who gave her the Edinburgh Scale test. I was with her when
she spoke to them. She might have answered the questions differently had she been on her own.

She said straight afterwards, 'Fancy them asking me if I felt
suicidal!'

She died just a few days later. She was 34 years old.

So much of Louise's story resonates with me, particularly
the deep sense of not wanting to be 'found out' by loved ones.
But I am also thinking of the other women who tragically died
or took their infants' lives despite being seen multiple times by
health professionals. How does this happen?

When I share the details of my own experience with Buist,
she tells me that my story, and my ability to hide what I was
going through so well, reminds her of a study conducted by Dr

Margaret Oates, one of the founders of perinatal psychiatry. 'Margaret Oates did a review of women who suicided postnatally,' Buist says. 'She found that a lot of them had had some contact with health professionals, but it had been missed quite substantially. That it had been downplayed by both patients and health professions as "just a bit of postnatal depression". She concluded that even the ones who hadn't been diagnosed with postpartum psychosis were in fact suffering from the condition. And there was a significant proportion of health professionals among this group.'

When I find the paper, the data is striking: mothers who took their own lives were relatively socially advantaged and well supported. Most had higher education, 'and a worrying number were health professionals'.

⌒

While I'm writing this chapter, the new *Australia's Mothers and Babies* report is released by the Australian Institute of Health and Welfare. Between 2011 and 2020, suicide was the third leading cause of death for mothers.

Looking at the data on maternal deaths, I'm interested in one detail: deaths are considered perinatal if they occur during pregnancy and up to forty-two days after the birth. Are we dramatically underestimating the true impact of maternal mental illness by using that cut-off? One group of Australian researchers certainly thinks so. Hannah Dahlen and her colleagues analysed late maternal deaths – those occurring between this forty-two-day cut-off and twelve months postpartum – between 2000 and 2006. Of the 129 deaths in this period, forty-eight were due to suicide or trauma (accidental injury, homicide or traffic accidents). Of the women who died by suicide, 73 per cent had a history of mental illness, substance abuse or both. Most of the women who died by accidental injury also had a history of mental illness or substance abuse.

Dahlen and her colleagues also found that deaths from suicide or trauma rose between nine and twelve months postpartum. This is important because, as the authors highlight, by this time post-natal services have all but dropped off. This period also coincides with women returning to the workforce, with some psychiatric services (including admission to MBUs and access to the PANDA helpline) ceasing at twelve months. As the authors noted in their conclusions, perinatal services are generally constructed to pro-vide short-term support. But this may not be enough. We need to be better at identifying those at risk of maternal suicide in their baby's first year – well beyond that six-week cut-off.

'Have you seen this?' It's the third time someone has sent me the article about Cynthia Wachenheim. Reading her story makes my insides churn. I can see myself so clearly in her experience – the helplessness, the hopelessness, the resolute belief that there was something deeply wrong with her baby that no else could see.

Her death terrifies me.

I need to get better.

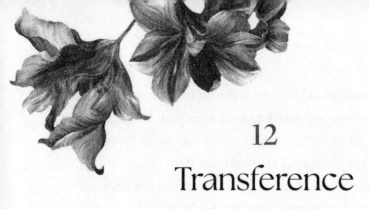

12

Transference

'We view all relationships through the lenses of early important relationships. At the same time, therapy can elicit especially raw feelings. This is because therapy is not just another relationship. It is an ongoing relationship between a person who may be in desperate need and a person who is there to provide help. The situation inherently stirs up powerful longings and dependency.'

DR JONATHON SHEDLER

Your doctor isn't supposed to fall in love with you. That should be the end of the sentence. But he does, this doctor. Somehow he falls for the broken mess you bring to his office week after week in the guts of your illness.

And you? How do you feel? It isn't love. It isn't. How could it be? But you are cared for and seen and hurting and he makes you hurt a little less. You have lost touch with reality and he has let you touch his. He has anchored you.

It won't make any sense for some time – years, in fact. You'll go over what happened, what was said, what was written. And what didn't happen, of course. Because he never touched you physically, and somehow that makes it even more confusing.

'I have become too emotionally involved in your care.'

But it's a mindfuck whichever way you look at it because he loved you, and he was supposed to look after you. You know this because he will tell you – in a way that you can never prove. Even writing that makes you sound crazy, doesn't it?

He is standing at the door of his office in a light-blue shirt. You have visited him here so many times over the past few months. It has been your safe place. He looks tired and sad and you're tired and sad and confused and unwell.

Really, deeply unwell.

You've been coming to see him regularly for about nine months, and that's how these things happen, right? You've studied psychology. You've read about Anna O and Breuer and Freud.

During those months, he listened while you cried. He shared pieces of music and poems and passages from favourite books he thought you might like. Once, before you leave his office, he scribbles 'Spiegel im Spiegel' by Arvo Pärt on a piece of paper, like a prescription. You've never heard it before and when you listen to it on the way home your feet are so firmly beneath you, so steady, because how you could you leave when something so exquisite exists? How could you possibly leave? He helped you stay.

You let him open you up, trusted him more than you trusted Dr Q. But why? He seemed to *get* you more than she did. He understood your urgency. He said he was going to fix you, said he'd try. And you believed him. You believed him because you had to believe there was a way back.

He helped you stay.

He went into your broken head, too fast, too fast, too soon, too deep. He wanted to help. You wanted him to help. But he was out of his depth.

'It appears roles have been blurred,' Dr Q will write. He is no longer part of your treating team.

∽

So how did it begin?

You and your husband have never had a completely traditional relationship, haven't always been completely monogamous. Your boundaries have always been more flexible. You have always been comfortable with grey. This detail shouldn't matter, you know this. But you wonder if somehow it does.

How do any of these things begin? The moving of boundaries ever so slightly. Letting you email. Letting you text. Making your appointments longer. The changing of the rules, the making you feel 'special'.

But you are not special.

'During a depression, the nature of transference and counter-transference, which naturally arises in all clinician and patient relationships, is more complex and more intense and therefore necessarily requires more careful negotiation,' Dr Q will write in a letter. 'This is not a time for any psychological exploration. In general, the nature of a depression is that it renders an individual more porous and able to access their premorbid core issues. Life events will naturally bring to the fore many existential issues, which cannot be objectively addressed in a melancholic state.'

'It feels like a break-up,' you tell Dr Q. 'It shouldn't feel like that.'

'It shouldn't feel like that,' she says. 'No.'

You are sitting in her chair, one cheek against the cool leather.

'It was transference,' Dr Q says.

'It felt real, though.'

'Yes,' she says gently. 'It was real transference.'

〜

You will write a poem and send it to Dr Q.

Poker-faced.
Cool detached scientist.
You collect your data.
Grope at her history; verbal foreplay.
You keep a practised distance.
But human.
All too human.
Your eyes hoard compassion you've rote learnt.

She is bleeding.
This is noted.
A clinical anomaly, a special case.
You read the inkblot of her words, with a hand wrapped around
her heart.
Diagnosis: Unconfirmed.
Prognosis: Unclear.

Unconditional. Without bounds.
She lies for you, face to a fluorescent ceiling.
You loom.
Godlike in white.
She has lost her way.
Might she have yours?
She almost believes you will give it to her.
You give so much.

You prescribe Beethoven, with your pills and words.
She listens. Dutiful student of recovery.
Why are you so kind to her?
You use words like 'worth' and 'intelligence'.
You don't say 'beauty'.
But you don't need to.
She sees herself burnt into your hassled eyes.
You carry her around like a locket.
She opens and closes for you.

You say she is weighted down with secrets.
That they define her, with the wrong words.
You say your definition is more accurate.
I think you know her better than she does.

One by one you extract them, coax, probe, prod.
They are delivered, bloody and screaming.
Ugly, speckled newborns.

You inspect them. Clinical voyeur.
Hold them up to the dark.
Weigh them.
They are not well.
Shrivelled with neglect.
Each cord is severed.
They suck the air from the room.

You keep them for her.
Tend to them.
Mould them.
And return them.

They are different.
They respond to your voice.
They are no longer hers.
She is without a past.
Disassembled.
You can't give her a new one.
You don't know how.

Crouched at my feet, small and needy,
you are as lost as I am.
I don't want your way.
Your way is wrong.
We have no compass.

I am still bleeding.
This is noted.
A clinical anomaly.
Your special case.
You read the inkblot of my blood.

And see your heart.

෴

You are slow again and can't remember if you exist. You take hundreds of photos of your feet just to prove that you're real. The heaviness is back.

In the shower one night you have a strange thought: *Even my skeleton is sad.* The bones holding you upright are fragile.

You are walking back from taking your baby to day care one morning when you step in front of a car. It beeps at you, brakes.

You see the driver's anger, hear the stress in his voice.
    He thinks it's a lapse of attention.
    You know that it's not.
    You go into hospital for the second time.

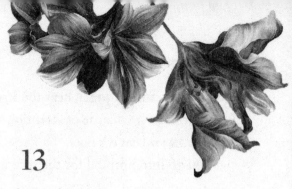

13

The Clock Test

*'I've been trying to write about the time I failed the
clock test but I can't find the words, like I couldn't find
the numbers or the hands, and I couldn't find my own
hands either or love or my heart and even though I
drew a full circle it was empty of time and the doctor
said it's okay sleep deprivation does strange things and
she gave me a new pill and a bingo from the DSM and
said time is a flat circle on a white bed beside an empty
clock and you are exactly when you need to be.'*

AUGUST 2021

*Thank you for considering Ariane for admission in the context of her
depressive illness, for the purposes of clinical review as well as a period
of rest and containment from the stressors and responsibilities in her
life at present.*

'Draw a clock, please,' the registrar says, 'and make the time 2.15.'

It's a standard part of the admission process to the mood disorder unit at a psychiatric ward on Sydney's North Shore, along
with all the usual questions about sleep and appetite, mood and

meds. I am in my room, sitting on the single white bed. Although I am back in hospital again, this time I will be alone – Henry is nearly two and mother and baby units only take babies up until they're twelve months old. This morning, I kissed him goodbye as we dropped him off at day care.

'We'll take care of him,' his favourite teacher tells me when I explain where I'm going. 'Go and get better, mama.'

I stare down at the blank piece of paper in front of me and draw a circle. I write the numbers 12, 1, 2, 3, 4, 5, 6, 5, 4, 3, 2, 1 and look at them, wondering why they don't make sense. I can't remember how to tell the time. The numbers swim in front of my eyes.

'I'm sorry,' I stammer, looking up at the registrar. She's wearing brown glasses and strong perfume. 'I can't seem to do it.'

'It's okay,' she says.

'But I don't understand …'

'Don't worry.' She smiles. 'We'll just move on. Sleep deprivation does strange things to us.'

As the registrar writes something in my file, I look over at Robb. He is ashen. Years later, he'll tell me that the clock test was the moment he really grasped how unwell I was. My broken brain was there, all over that piece of paper. I could no longer hide it.

At this stage, Ariane expresses a profound need to have some rest and reprieve from her stressors, which she has not been able to achieve at home or through her family support.

This hospital stay is a secret. The night before I go in, I send a message to Dad to tell him I'm being admitted, and could he please let Mum know? I text only a handful of people and say that I don't want any visitors, not this time. Somehow, being back in hospital feels like a deep, painful failure, even more than my admission to the MBU.

Not again. She's still sick? Isn't her kid, like, two?

'You don't have to go to bed,' a nurse says, when she checks on me an hour after I've been admitted. I am fully clothed, lying under the covers, facing the white wall.

'But I need to sleep,' I tell her. 'I'm not getting any sleep. I just need to sleep.'

'Oh, right, you're the mother,' she says, and closes the door.

Not long after, there's another knock. A nurse delivers my lunch, setting it down on the table beside me. I'd asked for a sandwich, and he looks me up and down as he hands it over.

'Perhaps you should have something a little more substantial tomorrow,' he says, pointing to the other options on the menu. 'You're very thin.'

'Okay,' I say, so he will leave me alone.

He nods and shuts the door.

Later, another nurse says, 'You don't have to smile.'

Treatment has been challenging with Ariane reporting sensitivity to most medication. Titration has been slow, particularly due to the sedation she experiences, and the need for her to be alert while taking care of her child.

'I take this medication at night,' I tell the nurse, when I collect my pills at the station before bed on my first night on the ward.

'The doctors have written that the Lexapro is for daytime,' she says.

'Oh, right.' I nod. 'Okay, but I've taken this at night for the last few months now, because it makes me really drowsy.'

The nurse almost throws the pill at me.

'Fine,' she snarls. 'Take it up with your doctor in the morning.'

Over recent months, while the severity of the melancholia has taken some time to improve, Ariane has also had to deal with several life events, resulting in grief and loss, including the suicide of her next-door neighbour and the death of a baby from her mother's group.

I climb into the single bed, fall in and out of restless sleep. I imagine the notes the nurses must be making about me. 'The Mother has chosen not to engage in group therapy. The Mother pretends to sleep during the day. The Mother can't tell the time. The Mother chose salad for lunch. Is very thin. Smiles too much. Could also be on the eating disorder wing. Was antagonistic towards nursing staff. Has boundary issues.'

The ward is full of much older men who leer at me when I walk past.

I don't leave my room unless I have to.

In the course of providing her support, Ariane was having regular appointments with myself and her GP as containment to prevent further isolation. From my understanding, exploration of her premorbid issues prematurely by her then GP resulted in worsening Ariane's mental state and adding to her distress.

'So you were doing some counselling with your GP?' asks the psychiatrist I'm assigned to during our first session. 'Is that right? Like therapy?'

'Yes. I suppose so. I was seeing him pretty regularly.'

'And did he ever touch you inappropriately?'

'Of course he didn't. Is that what the notes say?'

Consistent with her low mood, passive thoughts of not existing have been present, and more intensified during these periods of stress, but her relationship to both her husband and her son are protective factors.

'Oh, he's so cute,' a nurse squeals when Henry comes to visit me on my second night. 'Is he your little brother?'

Medication change and/or addition of other agents has already been discussed, but there has not been a clear opportunity to implement this in a period of stability, over the last few months.

The day before I am discharged from hospital, Robb is made redundant by Disney. His entire Sydney team will lose their jobs, and he's been tasked with telling them all, one after the other.

'Sorry,' Robb's boss tells him. 'We know the timing isn't great, mate. Anything we can do, just let us know.'

We're both unemployed.

Complicating this, Ariane has struggled with some of her premorbid core issues, and styles of dealing with challenges, which includes perfectionism, being particularly self-critical if not able to address a challenge, including not being able to return to work as quickly as she had hoped.

'Are you fucking kidding me?' I say, when Robb calls from the office to tell me about his redundancy. I am outside in the garden, where a group from the eating disorders unit are smoking. 'Can't we catch a break?'

'Look, it's not all bad,' Robb says. 'I'll be around for a bit now to help with Henry. Maybe it's a good thing.'

And while he's right, I am too depressed to share his optimism.

In addition to some reprieve for Ariane, I would appreciate your opinion or recommendations to optimise Ariane's psychiatric care.

'They gave me the afternoon off,' Robb says. 'I'll be there shortly.'
    'Least they could do.'

Yours sincerely,
Dr Q

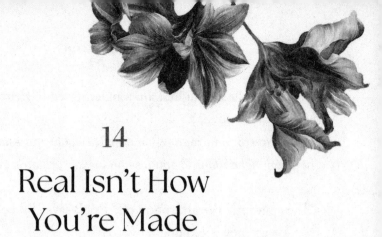

14

Real Isn't How You're Made

'Going mad takes time. Getting sane takes time.'

JEANETTE WINTERSON, *WHY BE HAPPY WHEN YOU COULD BE NORMAL?*

'I think you need a fresh start,' Dr Q tells me the first time I see her after leaving hospital. 'With someone new.'

'You don't want to treat me anymore?' I ask. My voice sounds whiny and small like a child's.

'That's not what I'm saying,' she says, leaning forward in her chair. 'I will stay on and look after your medication and the biology of your illness. But I think you need someone fresh to do psychotherapy. After what happened with Dr Wilson.' Dr Q pauses. 'What do you think?'

'I think I feel tossed between health professionals,' I sulk. 'I don't want to start all over again. I don't understand why you won't just see me for therapy.'

'Boundaries can be hard,' Dr Q says. 'But they're going to be important for your recovery.'

'Okay.'

'You tend to resist recommendations initially,' Dr Q says. That one's hard to argue with. 'We know this. It would be detrimental for me to collude with your old patterns.'

I let out a long sigh. 'Alright, then.'

⨪

Sandra, the psychologist I'm referred to through a clinician-matching service, groans when I tell her I'm also a psychologist. She's in her late fifties and gestures towards an empty chair next to a dehydrated pot plant.

'I'm not practising, though,' I say. 'Don't know if I ever will again.'

'And you have just the one child?'

'Yes. A boy.'

'I have boys,' she says. 'Two. Figured I should have a spare.'

'Yeah, right.' She doesn't see my eyebrow, arched to the stars.

Sandra prints off some Enya lyrics and gives me a worksheet about The Hero's Journey – Joseph Campbell's theory that all mythological stories share the same structure of a departure, an initiation and a return – to fill out before our next session.

'You said you like writing, didn't you?' she says.

'I did.'

'I think you'll find that exercise useful, then.' Sandra looks pleased with herself as she stands up. 'Let's complete this story together. Same time next week?'

'See you then.'

I return the following Wednesday, catching the train from Redfern to her small office in Sydney's inner-west, and again the week after. I am determined to be a Good Patient. But sharing my history feels less like the slow unravelling of a spool of thread, as it had with Dr Q, and more like hot wax being applied then stripped from my bruised psyche.

'You shouldn't still see yourself as a sick person,' Sandra tells me. 'You need to get past that.'

I've had better pep talks.

I keep going back.

During our fourth session, I tell Sandra that on the way to her office I saw myself falling onto the train tracks. The vision terrifies me – it has been some time since I've felt suicidal.

She inhales, shoulders back, and fixes me with a stare. 'And how do you think Robb and Henry would feel about that?'

I look at the clock above her desk. It's been seventeen minutes of our fifty-minute session.

'You know what?' I say, looping the strap of my handbag over my shoulder. 'I – I can't do this.' And it's so out of character, this rudeness, this assertiveness, that I laugh as I head to the door. 'This isn't going to work for me.'

Sandra leaps up and stands in front of the handle. 'I'm going to call Dr Q. I don't think you should leave while you're upset.'

'Call her,' I say. 'That's fine. But I would like to go, please.'

❦

While gathering papers for this book, I come across a list I'd made on the back of a page from the hospital manual.

2012

January – *First visit to GP. Diagnosed with PND. Prescribed Zoloft 25mg.*
March – *Saw psychiatrist on two occasions. Query of Bipolar 2. Suicidal ideation increased. Upped Zoloft to 50mg.*

April – *Admitted to SJOG. Withdrawn from Zoloft. Started Avanza 7.5mg. Discharged after 3 weeks. Avanza increased to 15mg.*
May – *Saw Dr Q. Psychotic depression. Withdrawn from Avanza. Medication-free for approximately six weeks.*
July – *Return to work two days per week.*
August – *Return of symptoms. Teary. Tired. Difficulty concentrating. Concerns around perception of/relationship with Henry. Am I real? Suicidal ideation. Commence Lexapro 10mg. Saw GP once a week, psychiatrist twice a week.*
September – *Commenced Seroquel 12.5mg.*
October – *Next-door neighbour's suicide. Symptoms remain. Teary, suicidal. Seroquel to 25mg.*
November – *Walked in front of car. Daily suicidal ideation.*
December – *Increased Lexapro to 20mg. Seroquel to 37.5mg. D's death.*
Jan/Feb – *GP.*
March – *Hospital.*

Reading this now, what strikes me is how tightly bound I was, even then, to orchestrating my own care. There's no emotion here – just the facts.

'I will take you on for psychotherapy,' Dr Q says to me, three days after my last session with Sandra. 'We will work hard. And there will be different rules.'

I nod.

'But you will have to let me steer the ship. 'Do you think you can let me do that?'

I am so hollow, so worn out, that I finally let her.

And we get to work.

ᔕ

203

We agree that I'm not well enough to go back to DoCS. I am useless. I have failed as a mother and now I can't return to a job I loved. I have failed as a psychologist too. I am completely and utterly financially dependent on my husband and the thought both terrifies and disgusts me.

On the higher dose of lamotrigine, my hair starts to fall out. Clumps of it block the drain when I'm in the shower.

'Let's reduce again,' Dr Q says. 'Taper down.'

Taper: to become progressively smaller towards one end.

'Have you read *The Velveteen Rabbit?*' Dr Q asks one afternoon, towards the end of our session. 'It's by Margery Williams.'

'I haven't, no,' I say. 'Should I?'

'It's a children's book,' she says, smiling. 'I think you'd like it.'

'Real isn't how you are made,' said the Skin Horse. 'It's a thing that happens to you. When a child loves you for a long, long time. Not just to play with, but REALLY loves you, then you become real.'

'Does it hurt?' asked the Rabbit.

'Sometimes,' said the Skin Horse, for he was always truthful.

Winnicott says we have a true self and a false self. 'Only the True Self can be creative and only the True Self can feel real,' he writes. 'Feeling real is more than existing; it is finding a way to exist as oneself, and to relate to objects as oneself and to have a self into which to retreat for relaxation.' A false self, however, develops when a baby's primary caregiver isn't able to adapt 'well enough' to the baby's demands (through illness, for example, or the demands of caring for other children). 'Where the mother cannot adapt well enough, the infant gets seduced into compliance and a compliant False Self reacts to environmental demands, and the infant seems to accept them.'

On the surface the concept seems easy enough to understand – and yet, while Winnicott's writings on good-enough motherhood, on breastfeeding and on play are often easy to follow, I find his explanation of how our false self develops frustratingly complex. It's not until I stumble across *Animal Joy* by poet and psychoanalyst Nuar Alsadir that it makes sense. Alsadir says that when a baby modifies its behaviour to please – something she calls a 'survival mechanism', given the baby's dependence on its caregiver – that's when the socialised self begins to develop. This socialised self is built around manners or protocols. 'Putting forward a False Self allows us to tuck away all the aspects of ourselves we don't want others to see, even if it means remaining silent, complicit or asleep.' We all have false selves, Alsadir explains. It's how we function in society.

> But a False Self that is so fortified by layers of compliant behaviour that it loses contact with raw impulses that characterise the True Self often results in a person feeing as though they don't really know who they are beyond what is signalled about their interior through the ideas, interests, friends and achievements they have accumulated from the outside world (imposter syndrome). When contact is made with the True Self, however, wires touch, switching on an inner light.

I have a very well-developed false self. I learnt to perform, to please, to shine, to be perfect. But I want to learn to be true. I am switching on that inner light.

Over our years together, Dr Q will say gently, but consistently, 'You don't feel real today. You are not in the room.' I am finding my way into the room. There are days when I am still finding my way into the room.

∽

My inability to cry doesn't happen immediately. Different medication has different side effects and perhaps, as I recover, I don't notice it straight away. When you've been depressed for so long, as feelings return, as the tears stop, it's a step forward.

Lying awake one night, I remember the artist who photographed what her tears looked like under a microscope. There were tears of grief, joy, sadness.

Has anyone looked at postpartum tears? I wonder. Half asleep, I grab my phone and do a Google search. The answers make me laugh and wince: 'Slide Show: Vaginal Tears in Childbirth'; 'Isolated Rectal Buttonhole Tears in Obstetrics: Case Series and Review of the Literature'; 'Perineal Tears, A Review'.

So, not quite the tears I was looking for. Perhaps I am guilty of trying to find the poetic where it simply doesn't exist.

But while no one has photographed postpartum tears, there's more to say on SSRIs and how they affect one's ability to cry. I find a journal article titled 'When I Want to Cry I Can't', which reports on seven cases of patients' 'inability to cry after treatment with selective serotonin re-uptake inhibitor (SSRI) medication, even during sad or distressing situations that would have normally initiated a crying episode'. As one patient says, 'It's like my body had forgotten how to cry. I try, but I can't.' In this case series, however, an inability to cry was associated with other 'inhibitory' side effects: in three patients, for example, sexual dysfunction was apparent.

But does it really matter if you can't cry? The authors note that while all patients had mentioned it to their doctors, the patients themselves didn't find it particularly distressing. The researchers thus concluded that not being able to cry isn't 'emotionally harmful'.

It may not be harmful, but oh how I miss the release of tears.

∾

Henry is too sick to go to day care and I am too unwell to miss my appointment with Dr Q. I take him with me on the train, one tired foot in front of the other. It's the first time they meet. Henry runs up the stairs and into Dr Q's office. I hand him my phone, preloaded with Fisher-Price apps, but he ignores it, taken with the novelty of this new space. He runs around the room, making it feel smaller than it ever has before, then climbs onto her chair and lies flat across the arm rest.

'Look, he's planking,' I say.

Dr Q opens her bottom drawer, pulls out a handful of chocolates. Henry toddles over, gobbles them down.

'Guess he made a miraculous recovery,' I sigh.

'Funny how they do that,' says Dr Q.

That evening, Dr Q emails: *Henry is lovely, and his comfort in the world is a credit to you both. I was glad to meet him.*

I'm thinking of her words later when I check in on Henry, who is sound asleep. I lie down next to his tiny body and feel its warmth. I am smitten. When the love eventually broke through the layers of depression, tearing at the numbness in my body and my mind, it didn't stop. It hasn't stopped.

'Do you remember when I asked if you wanted to bring Henry into one of your appointments?' says Dr Q. We are talking about the book and my early memories of our sessions. 'I think he was sick or something and you couldn't come in.'

'Oh yes,' I say, giggling. 'I was not … in favour.'

'You were not.'

'Do you remember what I said?'

'Not exactly, no. But I remember thinking you were worried I was going to be observing you with him. You didn't want to be observed.'

'I absolutely did not want to be observed.' I smile. 'I thought, "I know what she's doing. She wants to watch me. She wants to mark me on how good a mother I am."'

'I really didn't,' Dr Q says. 'I just didn't want you to miss your appointment.'

'Oh, I know that now.'

∽

I come across a *Psychology Today* article by Karen Kleiman called 'Holding Perinatal Women in Distress'.

> Your greatest task, as you share the sacred space with her pain, is to preserve the integrity of her wishes while you gently guide her toward a more complete state of well-being.
>
> You do this in spite of her resistance.
>
> You do this whether she believes she will get better or not.
>
> You do this to help her breathe whether she wants to be sitting there, or not.
>
> This is why she has summoned the strength to get dressed and be present in your office.
>
> My appeal to you is that you become comfortable with this paradox. You must refrain from seeking immediate solutions or quick fixes, (to reduce her anxiety or yours), you must sit, and wait, and embrace her suffering. In doing so, you set in motion the possibility of therapeutic engagement to take place.
>
> This is the essence of holding.

I email the link to Dr Q. 'You were holding me,' I write. 'The whole time. This is what you were doing.'

⁓

I'm dropping Henry at kindy one day when I notice a sign for a new ballet school, across the road in the church hall. I google it when I get home – during the day there are adult classes in RAD, the old Royal Academy of Dance syllabus I grew up with. I buy a leotard and a pair of black tights and go digging for the soft pink ballet shoes shoved up the back of my wardrobe.

There are two other students in the class when I arrive the following week. The teacher is young and trained in similar circles as I did, before she danced in the English National Ballet.

'Why didn't you dance professionally?' she asks me as I'm stretching afterwards. 'You're very good.'

'Too short,' I say. 'That was the main reason, anyway. And not thin enough, of course.'

She is small, too, but as we stand side by side we laugh – she's taller by only about 7 centimetres. Enough to change the course of a life.

Taking ballet for the first time in over a decade brings me back into my body and out of my head. In the studio, as my muscles recall the pirouettes, arabesques and pliés of my childhood, I remember who I was before I got sick, and I remember the sheer pleasure of movement.

'Dance until your bones clatter,' writes the poet Gabrielle Calvocoressi.

I clatter. I clatter.

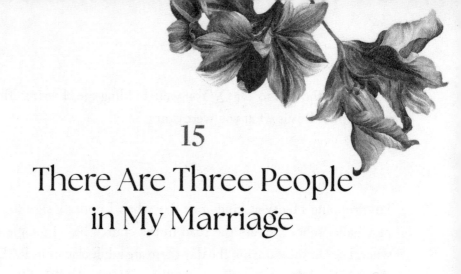

15

There Are Three People in My Marriage

'When you have a baby, you set off an explosion in your marriage, and when the dust settles, your marriage is different from what it was.'

NORA EPHRON, *HEARTBURN*

As I recover – slowly, ever so slowly – I am hungry for words again. When Henry was born, I packed away my books to make space for him. Robb lugged them up to the attic, box by box, mumbling under his breath about how many I own.

'You knew who I was when you married me,' I'd said, laughing.

But now we buy a bookshelf and I rescue some of my favour-ites from the attic: Drusilla Modjeska's *Poppy*, Gwen Harwood's *Collected Poems* and my forbidden Plath – poems, letters, diaries. I feel more like myself than I have in months.

It is, of course, not at all surprising that books about mother-hood are written by writers. Stay with me, though – I promise I have a point. While I had always enjoyed writing and dreamed of writing a book, when I became a mother and was unwell, I wasn't an author or even working as a writer. I found it difficult to relate to memoirs of women chasing grants and residencies, carving out time to write between naps and breastfeeds, or worrying they might never write again. I couldn't find myself in these stories and it was a lonely place to be.

And so, just as I had promised myself and the group on the mother and baby ward, I opened my laptop and I started to write.

ᔓ

'Thank you so much for sending this to *Mamamia*. We'd love to publish it. Would you like the post to run anonymously? Or are you happy for it to go with your by-line?'

When the email arrives, I run downstairs to where Robb is feeding Henry.

'They're publishing it!' I say, showing him the response from the deputy editor. 'My article!'

'That's amazing,' he says, grinning. 'But I knew they would.'

It's my first published piece, and when it goes live my heart hammers in my chest.

I find the piece hard to read even now. It is written from a place of pain, by someone who was still unwell but desperate to be seen.

For a time, Robb called my depression Prudence – a way of differentiating the recovering self from the depressed self. As I write in the article, Prudence is 'bad days personified'. 'There are three people in my marriage: me, my husband, and the woman my husband calls "Prudence". Prudence looks a lot like me. She sounds like me. And she's a mum. But the similarities end there.'

In many ways, it's the first time I have 'outed myself' beyond my close family and friends. It's my way of saying, 'This is where I've been, this is where I went, but I am on my way back now. I am on my way back.'

'I did not wilfully deceive them,' writes Susan Johnson, in her memoir *A Better Woman*, about sharing her own postpartum health challenges. 'It was just that I could hardly bear to have been such a failure at having a baby, an event in human life we know to be both ordinary and extraordinary but which we mostly take to be a commonplace.'

'I had no idea,' one of the day care fathers says. 'You always seem so happy.'

A school friend comments on Facebook. 'Aside from the courage it took to write this, I'm also very happy to see you're writing again! You were always writing something!'

I'm not well enough to be a psychologist, but maybe, just maybe, I can write.

ↀ

'I lost the woman I married,' Robb says over dinner recently. 'She never came back.'

'Yeah?' I ask.

'Yeah.'

'But this new version of me is better, right?'

'I love both versions of you,' Robb says with a laugh. 'But the new you is definitely more fun. There's a confidence you got through the rebuilding. That's the big difference.'

ↀ

'Daddy, am I real?' Henry asks Robb as they play on the floor. 'Or am I like the Lego people?' He holds up one of the small Lego figurines and pulls the head off, pinching it between his still-chubby fingers. Robb is momentarily stumped, then smiles and explains that yes, we are real, we have hearts and brains and feelings. Henry seems happy with the explanation and goes back to decapitating his Lego men, lining up the heads in macabre formation along the carpet.

'He's a bit young for an existential crisis, isn't he?' Robb jokes later. But I can tell he's pulled under in a way I haven't seen before. Triggers come in strange places.

I take photo after photo to prove that I'm real.

It's my turn to hold him.

While I had adjusted to life on the mother and baby unit – to psychiatric assessments, to medication doled out in tiny paper cups and sessions on mindfulness and CBT – Robb had to adjust, too. He and the other partners found themselves in the strange new role of 'carer', a bewildering and emotionally and physically exhausting reality as they juggled parenting and work and hospital visits.

I look at the MBU manual and come across the following line: 'It is not uncommon for partners of women with postnatal depression to experience some degree of depression or anxiety too. For this reason, we may ask partners to complete an Edinburgh Postnatal Depression questionnaire during the admission.'

I take a photo of the page and text it to Robb, asking if he remembers being assessed during my stay. 'Nope,' he replies. 'I think I got a tri-fold glossy pamphlet when we checked you out, from memory. A pat on the bum and a "Best of luck, champ". No one told me at the end of that what was ahead. No one said, "This isn't over yet."'

It's since changed the way he talks to the expectant and new dads in his life. 'I always say, "No one warns you that this stuff may even be an outside risk,"' he tells me over a wine. 'All the pre-natal warnings are about the baby. They drop one side note about "the baby blues may not be the baby blues". But it's lost in a sea of information about becoming a parent and this little being that you're about to be responsible for.

'So, you're focused on risks associated with the baby that you never really consider what the threat might be to your partner. Even if you do, it's likely to be physical things, not that you might take one woman to hospital and unknowingly leave with a com-pletely different person. And because none of this is on your threat radar, you can't possibly conceive how losing half your "team" will throw your collective lives into chaos for years.'

When he reads the first draft of this book, Robb sends me a screenshot of a quote from an earlier chapter: 'Our daughter took her own life suffering postpartum psychosis one week after deliv-ering her son. She was thirty-one and her first child. It happened so fast, we had no time or knowledge to seek help or an appropri-ate place to take her for help.'

'This is what I was trying to say,' he tells me. 'The speed at which it all happened. It's not at all gradual, it's upon you before you know what's happening. I couldn't articulate it until I read that. It all happened so quickly.'

We know from research that many couples struggle with the transition from partners to parents, and that their relationship satisfaction takes a massive dive. There are, of course, myriad rea-sons why this happens, but this quote from Esther Perel, from a panel with reproductive psychiatrist Dr Alexandra Sacks, cap-tures so much of this 'explosion'. 'Babies spell erotic disaster,' Perel says. 'Postpartum you have a different relationship to the body, to smell, to touch. Family life thrives on consistency, on routine, on repetition. Eroticism doesn't. It actually likes the mystery, the surprise, the unpredictable.'

And it's not just about sex, either.

When you become a caregiver, you sometimes begin to confuse offer and demand. So when your partner comes to you and wants to offer you a moment, an interlude, some connection, some play time, some chill, you think 'one more person that's coming to ask something from me'. Your partner is not coming to ask something from you. Your partner is coming to offer you something. Your partner is attending to a part of you that you at this moment are not able to pay attention to. Let the other person help you to not lose that part of you.

These are, of course, challenges all new parents face to varying degrees. But what happens when you add mental illness on top of an already stretched relationship?

'We never measured his height in the chaos,' Robb says to me out of the blue. 'That's something my parents did with me. You know, on the wall of the house? I regret that. It weighs on me. There was timber all over the fucking house. Why didn't I just do it? We were just so busy keeping the wheels on the wagon. We missed that stuff.'

Was Robb depressed? Most likely. Did anyone stop to check? Nope. But caring for an unwell wife and a new baby while trying to keep his career going left him a shell, from which it also took years to recover. I am conscious, too, of how much my illness affected his career. There are countries we missed out on living in, roles he couldn't take because I simply wasn't well enough to be uprooted – and because we prioritised stability for Henry after years of choppy waters.

I carry the guilt of this – among so many other guilts. But we are still together – we are still together.

⁊

A few years ago, a large study caught my eye. A team of researchers had examined the impact of what they called postpartum psychiatric episodes on the probability of divorce. The Danish study, published in *The Journal of Clinical Psychiatry*, found that in a sample of 266,771 new mothers, those diagnosed with a postpartum mental health condition had a higher probability of divorce in the years following their diagnosis than mothers who did not. And the more severe the illness, the more likely they were to divorce.

While the focus of this book has been on mothers and birthing parents, it's imperative to recognise that partners can be affected by perinatal mental illness, too. It is estimated that one in ten fathers will experience anxiety and/or depression in the perinatal period. Fathers and partners can also experience birth trauma and PTSD. And – like mothers – fathers and partners should also be screened for perinatal anxiety and depression and referred for treatment and support.

If you know someone experiencing perinatal mental illness, make sure you also check in on their partner. Their heart needs holding, too.

⁊

'Dr Q says I need a hobby,' I tell Robb one afternoon after our session. 'She suggested pottery.'

Robb snorts. 'You? Doing pottery?'

'That's what I said. But she's worried about me having too much time to think. And she reckons I need to do something that's not cognitive like writing, and not something I'm good at like dancing.'

'Right. Fair enough.'

'I suggested taking a lover.'

'Oh yeah?' Robb says, not looking up from his laptop. 'And what are her thoughts on that?'

As well as finding a hobby, Dr Q suggests we see a couples' counsellor. We leave Henry with Evan and catch a cab into the city. The office is down a long flight of steps. We sit on a couch opposite a man in his fifties.

'So what brings you here?'

I don't remember what we talked about. I've no doubt I presented our 'case' with aplomb. But I do remember how it felt – as though we were taking a deep breath in together and exhaling, both our stories filling the room in all the ways they were different and all the ways they were the same.

By the end of the session the counsellor has said very little, just asked a few probing questions, and Robb is holding my hand and we're smiling because holy shit all of that really happened and when you say it all like that in one gritty go, we're doing pretty well.

And that's exactly what the therapist says as he leads us to the door. 'Take care of one another. But if you'd like to come back, please do.'

We walk out into the night, together, laughing.

⌒

'Start organising the strippers! We're engaged!'

When Brooke's boyfriend asks her to marry him, I assume that I'll be one of her bridesmaids. We've been friends for so long and she's the one person I really let in at my lowest. She visited me both times in hospital – even the second admission, when I didn't want to see anyone, when even family were told to stay away.

When I realise that I'm not a bridesmaid, it hurts more than I want to admit. It's embarrassing, but I am gutted. I lash out. I send long messages going around in hurtful circles. I am not myself, but it's no excuse. I behave badly.

Nora Ephron was right about babies and marriage and how different things are after the dust settles, but what I didn't realise was just how much my friendships would change, too. I am not blameless – something Robb firmly but kindly reminds me of often. My friends tried so hard when I was unwell. They really did. They didn't give up on me; I gave up on them. Many of them couldn't have tried any harder. But the saddest thing is that I don't think I could have either.

How do you explain to someone that the little energy I did have I gave to Henry? He ate up the smiles I was able to muster, and the nursery rhymes I sang with a quivering voice.

Reassessing my friendship with Brooke and how much it has changed makes me realise that as I hunkered down and focused on my family, venturing out to see my psychiatrist once a week, the world continued without me. And while I was treading mud in a present I thought would never end, my friends – understandably – were moving on with their lives.

Women often talk about losing friends when becoming mothers. It's hard enough to maintain friendships when you're knee-deep in nappies and sleep deprivation – and even harder when you're a new mum and severely depressed.

In the years since I had Henry, the years where my friends

began to have children, many have reached out to say, 'I'm finding this so hard. I don't know how you did it while so unwell.'

And the thing is, you can't know until you *know*.

I know that now.

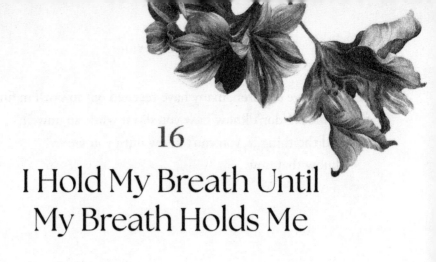

16

I Hold My Breath Until My Breath Holds Me

'When are you having a second baby?'
EVERYONE

When the mums from my mothers' group begin giving birth to their second children, my fingers itch to hold them. I revel in their newborn scent and drink in their perfect tiny features. The idea of having another of my own, however, fills me with terror. No, that's too soft – it fills me with horror.

It isn't until Henry turns three and all the babies start turning one that I feel a sense of grief.

'This is my baby,' one of his friends says to me one morning at day care drop-off. His little brother, who has the same eyes but chubbier cheeks, grins up at me from his pram. 'Where's your baby?'

I laugh and gesture to Henry. 'He's my baby,' I say.

'No, I'm not, Mummy, I'm a big boy,' Henry insists as he runs off to join his buddies.

And it hits me that he is.

For the first time, I feel primal rumblings. I find myself resting my hand on my stomach, a habitual gesture left over from pregnancy. My ovaries ache in the presence of newborns. And yet I am not ready psychologically.

I meet my niece, Jacqui's third baby. I am cradling her in my arms when I see myself fly out of my body and over my head. I watch myself move across the sky, over the trampoline and swimming pool in their Brisbane backyard. I hand the baby back to Robb, who is sitting beside me with his dad. It is as though I am watching my own madness, it is happening before me *and* to me simultaneously.

I am still not ready.

During a session with Dr Q, I ask about my medication as I'm struggling with side effects again. I wonder out loud if I'll always need to take them.

'Well, if you were ever thinking of having another baby,' she says, 'then we'd take you off the —'

'Don't rush me, Dr Q,' I snap. 'No one else seems to be pressuring me but you.'

She pauses. The outburst is unusual.

'I'm sorry,' I say. 'I didn't mean that.'

Second baby announcements are the hardest. I am part of the first baby club – I am not part of the second. I feel a fresh wave of grief each time a friend or family member shares baby news, and the shame that follows the guilt.

For years, I believe every month that I am pregnant, and every month before my period arrives I panic. I check my breasts for the river of blue veins – the first sign I recognised before the positive test.

Every month, the relief of blood is immense. Every month, I breathe out.

Robb, too, is traumatised. 'My biggest fear was going through it again,' he tells me. 'If you got as sick as you got the previous time, what would that mean for us? How would we survive that? I was so scared of that.'

What does recovery from perinatal mental illness mean? What does it look like? How do you know when you're ready for another baby? Research shows that if you experienced postnatal depression with your first pregnancy, you're likely to experience it again. A study of 450,000 Dutch mothers showed that, when compared with mums who didn't experience PND after their first baby, those who were diagnosed and treated with antidepressants were twenty-seven times more likely to experience it again. And if, like me, you were hospitalised with PND, you are forty-six times more likely to have it again.

When it comes to postnatal psychosis, one episode increases a mum's chance of it happening again to about 50 per cent. However, according to the UK's Royal College of Psychiatrists, there's a good chance that any further psychiatric episodes won't be linked to having another child. 'Avoiding having further babies does not guarantee that you will stay well.'

'Do you think this is odd wording?' I text Robb. '"Avoiding having further babies"?'

'Could be better, yeah.'

Over the years, people have said, 'But it would be different the second time. Everyone would be watching you and you'd put supports in place.' And I know, have always known, that rationally, yes, that's true. Dr Q would be there, and I'd have medication and experience and insight. No one would let me fall.

But it's not quite that simple.

~

Henry asks me, 'Does your body make the decision to have another baby, or do you?'

While he plays with his toys, I hold my breath until my breath holds me.

'It takes a long time to make a baby,' he continues. 'Maybe that's why it's taking a long time.'

Water rises in my eyes, just water because the drugs take the ache but also the tears. (Is that better or is that worse?) I don't know what to do with this grief that isn't a loss of something but a loss of nothing, because can you lose something you never had?

'You need a strong body to have a baby,' Henry says.

'You do, my darling,' I say. 'You do.'

And I look down at the limbs that carry me, that carried him, and I want to say that my body is strong, my body is willing. It's my mind that's fragile.

But I am working on making it strong. I am building it like a muscle and one day it will be as strong as my body, as strong as my heart.

∽

We plan for a second. Henry is four years old, so will be at school when the baby arrives. But just weeks after beginning to taper my medication, Robb is made redundant once again from the start-up he's been managing for the past two years. The business has been acquired and the Australian office has been written out of their plans. It's the second redundancy in four years. We sell our car to pay the mortgage.

With the sudden closure of the office, our small living room fills with boxes and ten 27-inch screens. It is claustrophobic and my mental health takes a dive. Being so ill again is a shock. The heaviness and lethargy come back, as well as the feeling of being suspended somewhere between consciousness and unconsciousness. I can't read or write. I am overcome with the familiar desire to hide away, to isolate myself, to conserve energy from all non-essential aspects of my life. I am back in survival mode.

Parenting through depression with a newborn is very different to having a preschooler. Four-year-olds demand attention. They need information, discipline, boundaries, consistency. They talk and talk and talk. There are days when Henry's constant chatter reverberates around my skull. If I try to rest on the lounge while he plays, Henry grabs my hand and pulls me upright. Long pram walks are replaced by trips to the park, requests for food and water and a turn on the swing – and small talk with other parents, when all I crave is silence.

But the biggest difference is our relationship and how much it helps me get well. Our bond grew when he was a newborn, but my love for Henry during this depression is fierce. And although parenting leaves me exhausted, Henry punctuates our days with magic and light.

But the relapse is a wake-up call. And I listen to it.

Much of what Winnicott had to say about mothers and babies is timeless. His writing in *The Only Child*, however, probably isn't his best work.

> When there are no children available there can be dogs and other pets, and there are nursery schools and kindergartens. If the immense disadvantages of being an only child are understood, they can be got round to some extent, provided the will to get round them exists.

Facebook history reminds me of a status from when Henry was five: *Henry: Mum you can't drink wine if you have a baby in your tummy because babies can't drink wine. If we get a cat though ... You can drink wine.*

We get a cat.

⁓

'I don't think I can do this,' I tell Dr Q. I am sitting on the leather chair in her office.

'Do what?' she asks.

'Have another baby.'

'You don't have to.'

'I don't think I can,' I say. 'But I also don't think I want to.'

'That can't be easy to admit.'

'It's not.'

There are tears now because there's relief and grief and relief and grief and exhaustion.

We increase my medication back up to where it was.

I'm still not ready.

Recovery from severe mental illness doesn't happen in a neat line. There are spirals downwards, leaps forwards. Long stretches of 'good days' are punctuated with heart-achingly bad ones that leave you wondering if you'll ever be completely well.

As the months – and years – roll by, there's never a time when I feel 'ready'. There's never a moment when I think, *It's okay, it's time. I can take my battered brain and the trauma that still lives in my blood and skin, and I can try to do this again and do it better.* The moment never arrives.

'You should have another one,' a woman – a stranger – says to me at an event, while I tell her about my seven-year-old son. 'He'll be lonely.'

The words sting, then burn. My head is full of champagne and the room is crowded, so I smile – a weary, polite, reflex of a smile.

'Maybe,' I mumble. 'We'll see.'

But she doesn't stop.

'You're still young! You should have another.' There's a pause. 'So he's not lonely.'

I take another swig of champagne. 'Why don't you mind your own business and not tell me what to do with my bloody uterus?' I respond.

Except I don't. Instead, I feel the familiar pinpricks of guilt, the feelings that arise whenever the 'only child' question comes up. My mood deflates and with it my heart. For this isn't an isolated incident – it happens often. And I am tired, so very tired of it.

'Becoming a mother almost killed me,' I want to say. 'There's no way to sugar-coat that. Postnatal psychosis tore my mind apart, leaving me aching to die at the same time as I welcomed a brand-new life. The cruelty of it, of this maddening juxtaposition, still makes me want to weep for all I lost to this frightening, horrific time. The trauma is softer now. It's not as raw and sharp, and it doesn't engulf me when triggers threaten to pull me under.

'But let me be clear: it's taken seven years to get to this point. This health, this happiness, is hard-won. And I don't want to, can't risk, losing it again. I am here, alive, well – and mother to a little boy whose resilience and humour and intelligence take my breath away. He needs me more than he needs a sibling. So, with respect: back off.'

ᔕ

On the day my sister, Lulu, has her third baby – a girl – Evan and Amy discover they're to have a son, their second child after their daughter. In the flurry of happiness, tears and my own cracked heart, I accidentally send my sister a 'Congratulations on your new baby boy!' gift pack. I don't realise the error until I see the receipt.

'I'm so sorry,' I text her. 'I am such a dickhead.'

'Don't be stupid,' she replies. 'The teddy is very cute. And we're shocked she wasn't a boy too.'

That night, my mum calls to see how I am. I cry so hard I can't speak.

She starts to cry, too.

'You really don't think you could have another?' she asks. 'I'd drop everything to help.'

'No,' I say. 'I really can't.'

Later, my mum texts me: 'I feel intensely, physically and emotionally, the ache and the pain … that your birth experience was so so traumatic for you … and that you've been denied another experience of pregnancy. I'm so proud that I now see the strong, beautiful daughter I gave birth to 37 years ago who filled my world with the utmost joy, a rapturous moment I will never forget.'

Thinking about Henry not having a sibling is painful. I would not be who I am without Evan, Lulu and Huw. And though we fight and bicker and roast one another, though we're as different as we are similar, I would do anything for them – and they for me. Evan and I have always been particularly close, and it was him (and his partner, Amy) who perhaps saw me most clearly when I was struggling, continuing to just show up even though he wasn't sure what was going on.

He's the one I text crying when Henry tells me one day: 'I just realised I won't be an uncle.' He's the one who understands the pain of this the most as he loves being an uncle to my boy.

My siblings remind me of what Henry is missing out on and this breaks my heart. But every day Henry heals it, too.

These signs of healing are everywhere. When Lizzie has her second baby, I visit her in hospital with a bottle of wine and a box of sushi. Robb drives me to the maternity ward and we catch the lift up together. As he reaches for my hand, my heart beats faster. I couldn't do this last time. Now, I can't wait. When we reach her room, Lizzie is sitting with her husband and has ice packs under her arms. Her new baby is fast asleep in the clear crib beside her.

'I have quad boobs,' she says, raising one of her arms up. 'See?'

'You have what?' I ask.

'Two extra boobs,' she says. 'Four boobs. It happens when I have a baby. They have nipples, and they lactate and everything.'

'Seriously?'

'Yep.'

She starts laughing and I'm laughing so hard I almost wake her newborn daughter. When she does stir, I sit and hold her, breathing in her new-baby smell.

For the first time, it doesn't hurt.

∽

When women struggle with motherhood, I feel an instant need to swoop in and protect them. When they don't, I often feel jealous, envious that their experience wasn't as terrible as mine. I feel like a monster even thinking this, but it's true.

I will be thirty-nine soon and my biological clock isn't ticking so much as screeching.

During my preschool ballet class one morning, I watch the baby sister of one of my students wiggling her legs along with the music. Her eyes follow her older brother as he darts around the room, waving the moon wands we're using.

Just because my mind has decided not to have more children, it doesn't mean that my body has received the memo. And yet, even though Robb offers to have a vasectomy, I still can't close that door. The body is willing, but the mind is not.

I let them continue their battle.

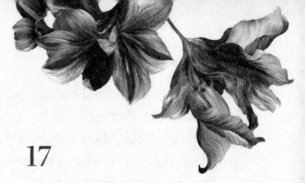

17

The Year My Brain Broke

'*When a woman tells the truth she is creating the possibility for more truth around her.*'

ADRIENNE RICH

'The Year My Brain Broke', an article I write for *The Sydney Morning Herald*, pours out of me, almost ready-made. The piece goes live
with a photo of me and Henry smiling. It's the most vulnerable
and raw article I've written so far – and the first time I've spoken
about being a mental health professional with a mental illness.

My editor, the lovely Natalie, handles it with care and compassion. 'I had a similar experience!' she tells me. In her, I find an
ally in the strange world of media – a world I do not yet understand. While I had always wanted to be a writer, I did not expect
to ever find myself in a newsroom.

I watch the Facebook comments roll in and the number of
retweets grow. It's both overwhelming and exhilarating. I feel
deeply exposed. An account on Twitter, @EndMedicalAbuse,
quote tweets my article. 'And again, all this speaks to is the them
and us attitude of MH health professionals. I wonder what she
was like before she had a breakdown, with the ppl who were not
"well".'

The message punctures me. I break down in the Fairfax multi-faith room, a small space next to the busy newsroom. Because I don't cry very often anymore, thanks to the SSRIs, once the tears start they don't stop. Everyone has been so kind and encouraging and the weight of seven years of grief and pain and battle and luck and love and hope is at once too much. I cry until my lungs ache.

As I'm about to return to my desk, my colleague Michael comes by.

'You okay?'

'Nope.'

'Come on.' He waits with me while I howl again, doubled over and breathless.

'Fuck, that felt good,' I say, laughing when there are no tears left.

'A similar thing happened when I wrote about my sister's death for the first time,' Michael tells me. 'It's no small thing, being so honest. And the grief can take you by surprise.'

It is no small thing.

I wipe my eyes and redo my ponytail.

'You going to be okay?' Michael asks.

'Yeah.' I smile. 'I am.'

Later that evening, there's a Facebook message from a friend: 'Your piece was shared on the national provisional psychologists' Facebook page,' he writes. 'It prompted lots of people to discuss their difficulties with receiving appropriate mental health care while practising or training to practise.' The writer Andrew Solomon shares my piece on social media, as does a neuroscientist I admire and follow on Twitter. My inbox fills with messages from other health professionals – many of whom are not yet 'out' about their own mental illnesses. I feel useful for the first time in months.

The following week I see a Facebook post by the Centre of Perinatal Excellence (COPE) asking for volunteers. Something about publishing the article, the final piece in my story, has given me a renewed sense of purpose, drive and closure. Might there be a place in this sector for me? I message COPE and am surprised when its founder and executive director, Dr Nicole Highet, responds almost immediately. Her enthusiasm is palpable and when she calls me the next day, we speak for almost two hours.

During our conversation, I learn that after thirteen years at Beyond Blue, Dr Highet founded COPE following the growth of Australia's National Perinatal Depression Initiative (NPDI). The $85-million initiative, which ran from 2008 to 2013, was a national approach to promoting, preventing, identifying and treating women at risk of or experiencing perinatal mental illness. COPE was established out of the NPDI's recommendation for a centre of excellence to provide a national focus for perinatal mental health in Australia.

I tell her about my own experience, how long it's taken to feel well again. And how much I'd like to help if I can.

I offer to do some volunteer work – writing blog posts and promoting the charity's annual fundraiser. Two months later, Dr Highet offers me a job managing COPE's social media accounts. The role will fit around my job at Fairfax and let me dip my feet, tentatively, back into mental health.

It's a new beginning – and it feels perfect.

❧

Less than a year after the Nine–Fairfax merger, our small team at *Essential Baby* and *Essential Kids* move from the *Sydney Morning Herald* newsroom to Nine. At the time, the businesses were in two different offices in Wharf 10 at Pyrmont. Our new colleagues are *Wide World of Sports*, digital 9News and *9Honey*.

My maiden article at Nine is 'Zeta-Jones' Instagram Shock' – 400 words about the moment actress Catherine Zeta-Jones discovered via social media that her son, Dylan, had been skydiving. 'Don't tell mum,' Dylan wrote on Instagram, where he shared footage of his skydive. 'Mum just found out,' Zeta-Jones wrote underneath, along with a healthy dose of unimpressed emojis.

We're taught to use strong emotive language, such as 'mumshame' and 'backlash', in our headlines, and which celebrities get clicks and which don't. (Chrissy Teigen is in, the Kardashians are out; this is always subject to change.)

It's a very different environment to the Fairfax newsroom, and I struggle to find my place and my people. We're no longer able to write about baby announcements (that's *Honey Celeb*) or the royal kids (that's *Honey Royal*). Sponsorships mean that articles like 'Mums Go Off Their Rocker for New ALDI Nursing Chair' (yes, that's a real headline I once wrote) make it harder to navigate what we can and can't write about.

I start to wonder what on earth I'm doing.

At 4.25 p.m. on one particularly difficult day, I call it and decide to head home. I grab my bag and struggle to open the door to the new office – a push-not-pull situation. Outside, standing by the lift, is a man I haven't seen before. He has kind eyes and is wearing a crumpled shirt, half tucked in.

'You're from *Essential*,' he says. 'I'm sorry we haven't met yet.'

'Yes, I'm Ariane,' I say.

'How are you finding it?'

'A little tough, actually,' I say with a sigh, all fucks gone.

'Oh yeah?

'Yeah.'

'Is it very different from Fairfax?'

'Totally,' I say, grateful for a receptive ear. 'I'm writing a lot of tragedy porn, for example. Lots of churns from *The Sun* about sick children. I wrote a piece that was really important to me and when I checked the home page, the headline was just terrible. I felt so bad, but I don't even know who I ask to get it changed. It's terrible, though. I'm so embarrassed.'

My new friend pulls his phone out and scrolls down.

'Killer bug?' he says, deadpan.

'That's the one.'

'Right. Leave it with me. I'll let them know to change it.' He types something on his phone then looks up again. 'Look, I get it. I do. Just keep telling good stories,' he says. 'You'll be okay.'

'Thank you,' I say. 'It's just a big adjustment.'

'Yeah, I know.'

'Sorry, I didn't catch your name.'

'Oh, sorry,' he says. 'I'm Jay, one of the editors.'

Shit. Of course you are.

Later that night I send Jay an email, thanking him for his time and apologising for my inappropriate language and lack of filter.

'I love no filter,' he fires back. 'You'll fit right in.'

But even though I try, I never really do.

～

'Do you think I'm more at risk of a psychotic break at the moment?' I text Dr Q. It is April and Australia is in its first lockdown of the Covid-19 pandemic. 'I feel untethered to time, like when Hen was a newborn.'

Dr Q, whom I haven't seen in the weeks since we went into lockdown, organises a telehealth consult the next day.

'Does that work?' she texts back. 'If you need to go to emergency then I understand, rather than wait until tomorrow.'

'Hold up. Robb just spilt red wine everywhere. Henry said, "It looks like someone died in here." I'm okay. Just really exhausted and not sleeping well.'

'Take your time.'

'Okay, let's talk tomorrow.'

I am not the only one who draws comparisons between lockdown and the newborn bubble. The minutes, hours, days all blur together. But I don't have a newborn. Instead, I am working full-time – three days at *Essential Baby* and two days in perinatal mental health with COPE – as well as supervising Henry's Year 3 homeschooling. He is eight years old – a funny, dancing, football-playing delight who doesn't understand why he can't see his friends.

At Nine I write articles about Covid and pregnancy, Covid and kids, Covid and changes to antenatal care. At COPE, I write web pages and emails about managing anxiety around Covid, finding online villages in the absence of mothers' groups and how to sit with so much grief. And I answer messages from panicked mums who are worried they won't be allowed to have a support person while giving birth.

'We must remain aware that pregnancy and parenting are associated with anxiety and depression and that the current environment will only exacerbate this risk for women, their partners, and families,' notes the Royal Australian and New Zealand College of Obstetrician and Gynaecologists (RANZCOG) in March 2020.

We don't know it yet, but it's just the beginning.

$\backsim$

As the pandemic continues and the pressures on expectant and new parents intensify, I wonder if the same might be the case for postpartum psychosis. Might we see an increase in cases of psychosis, too? I find a case series of three Indian women with asymptomatic Covid-19 published in the *Asian Journal of Psychiatry*. All developed postnatal psychosis within seven days of giving birth and two had delusions around Covid itself. One mother believed that doctors and nurses were trying to make her and her baby Covid-positive, despite already knowing she had tested positive; another believed she was being blamed as a Covid spreader.

In a paper published in *Archives of Women's Mental Health*, Dr Jessica Coker and her colleague Dr Erin Bider report on a similar phenomenon. After noticing an increase in cases of postnatal psychosis at the Women's Mental Health Program at the University of Arkansas for Medical Sciences, they looked at the data. They were right: between March 2020 and February 2021, nine women were diagnosed and treated for postnatal psychosis, compared with an average of 2.2 women per year in the preceding five years. Three of the women had Covid, while one had not been infected but had received the vaccine. The authors theorised that the pandemic appeared to be a risk factor for postnatal psychosis, regardless of whether the mum had had Covid, due to isolation exacerbating what is already a stressful time.

And it is a stressful time for so many of us. I am homeschooling and working – juggling like so many other parents across Australia, across the world – when I see the Circle of Security again playing out in my living room.

Watch over me
Delight in me

Help me
Enjoy with me

Hen is in Year 4 and he's normally quite independent and happy to amuse himself, but more recently he's hovered close. One morning, as I try to respond to emails, he decides to build a house for the cat out of cardboard boxes (sunroof included). He narrates as he goes, and I'm reminded of his preschool years, of being peppered with questions (300 per day, according to research) and the contents of his inner monologue.

Another morning, he crashes the adult ballet class I'm teaching via Zoom and does pas de deux with the cat. How not to be delighted? But I'm aware of how small his circle is – how much he needs me. When class is over, I call out for him to come downstairs.

'Want to ditch school this afternoon and watch a movie?'

Later that evening, I text to Lizzie, 'Pick a feeling.' She's now the mother of three young kids and holding the fort while her husband finishes his medical training.

She replies, 'On my hands and knees, crawling to the finish line this week. You?'

'Screaming inside my heart.'

୶

It's not long before about 70 per cent of my stories are coming courtesy of Reddit's Am I the Asshole (AITA) thread.

AITA because I didn't replace the blouse my baby spewed on? AITA for breastfeeding my sister's baby? AITA for having a spycam set up on my nanny? AITA for not wanting to name my baby after my boyfriend's ex-wife?

'I'm Nine's chief AITA correspondent,' I tell Paul one day.

'Is there a Walkley category for that?' he asks. Since returning from Oxford with a doctorate, he's now working as an expert in Indigenous child protection. Our jobs couldn't be more different.

By mid-2020, the entire newsroom is working from home. I haven't been into the office for weeks. My editor sends me a message on Slack: 'Can you do the "Cat got me pregnant" one before the Covid one, please? They want it for the lunchtime traffic.'

I send the message to Robb and Evan.

'Dream job,' says Robb.

'Capitalism blows,' says Evan.

'I reckon I'm done,' I say.

I resign a few weeks later to work full-time for COPE and to teach dance – my first love – at a studio in Sydney's inner west. Rediscovering ballet has been healing, particularly as an adult, when the strict rules of the classroom no longer apply. And teaching beginner adults is both a thrill and a joy. In my classroom, there are the portable barres and mirrors and classical music from my childhood, but there's laughter and camaraderie and cheers when a fellow dancer masters a tricky step or when a piece of choreography falls into place. And, as I discover, there's the beauty of imperfection – the unbridled freedom of it.

I clatter, I clatter.

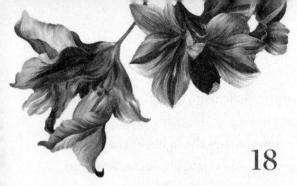

18

Well, What Do You Expect?

'We did not entirely understand that Mother, as
imagined and politicised by the Societal System,
was a delusion. The world loved the delusion more
than it loved the mother.'

DEBORAH LEVY, *THINGS I DON'T WANT TO KNOW*

It's one a.m. on 12 June 2021 when a new mum, Melinda, calls an
ambulance to her home in regional NSW. Since giving birth to
her first baby, a daughter, she has felt her grip on reality loosen.
She's disoriented, wired, high, feels as though her body is failing
her. And now her thoughts have turned darker.

The paramedics, a young man and a young woman, are dis-
missive – they tell Melinda to seek more support from her family,
join a playgroup or try bottle-feeding. But she's already been to
her GP, called the Australian Breastfeeding Association. Her calls
to a number of other helplines have been met with answering
machines.

The female paramedic takes Melinda to the ambulance, where
she checks Melinda's heart rate. The male paramedic tells her

husband, Simon, who is cradling their baby, that they'll let him know what's happening. But they don't. Instead, sitting on the couch with their daughter, Simon watches the lights of the ambulance disappear down the driveway. He's left behind, anxious and distressed, with a baby who is solely breastfed. Melinda's phone battery has gone flat.

There's no breast pump at Casino Hospital and so, after receiving a frantic phone call from Simon, Melinda's mother-in-law drives her to Lismore Base, another hospital nearby. Ever since her milk came in, Melinda has had an oversupply, with several bouts of undiagnosed mastitis. She is in constant pain. A few nights prior, after feeding her baby, a waterfall of milk had poured down the side of the bassinet. She was petrified she had almost drowned her baby. By now, Melinda's breasts are engorged and she is in agony.

It's four a.m. when they arrive at the second hospital. The harried emergency registrar barks at her, 'Tell me your story.' So she does, again, starting with an induction, an emergency C-section in a too-bright theatre, a baby placed on her chest, and a body entering fight or flight. By now, three and a half months post-birth, Melinda has presented to hospital five times in seven days with panic attacks, intrusive thoughts and paralysing anxiety. She feels manic, hypervigilant, fractured. She doesn't feel safe in her own body.

But the doctor is abrupt.

'Well, what do you expect?' he says. 'What do you want me to do about it? It's four o'clock in the morning. Our mental health-care team has gone.' Exhausted, Melinda struggles to string her words together. This only frustrates the doctor further. He asks her if she's tried the community nurse and Tresillian. She has. She's still suffering.

Melinda pleads to be admitted to the women's care ward and for a breast pump.

'They're busy up there,' the doctor says. 'And it's for new mothers and babies only.'

She pleads again.

'Look,' he says, reluctantly. 'I'll see what I can do.'

A midwife comes down to ED and assists Melinda to express her milk.

'You should be grateful,' the doctor says.

Distraught and feeling ignored, Melinda decides to head home. What she doesn't know, but will later find out when she accesses her records, is that someone from mental health was on their way to see her. Melinda has already left when they arrive.

Back at home, Melinda has another panic attack and flashbacks from her traumatic birth. She's afraid to be left alone. Increasingly desperate and suicidal, Melinda returns to Casino Hospital, where she waits to be seen for eight hours. This time she grabs hold of a nurse's arm. This time she begs. 'I feel like if I fall asleep, I might die.' This time, they listen.

'You're entering psychosis,' a mental health nurse says. 'We need to get you off this roundabout.' But with no mother and baby unit nearby, Melinda's options for treatment are limited. She is sent back to Lismore Hospital where, after another two-hour wait, she is discharged with medication and the promise of a visit from the local mental health team.

At home, Melinda sleeps for four hours straight – the first sleep she's had in three days. The two mental health workers who arrive the next morning are kind and softly spoken.

'We've got you and we will not let you slip through the cracks again,' they tell her. 'We've got you.'

She finally believes them.

✧

I first meet Melinda over Zoom after messaging back and forth for weeks. I had heard about her petition to the NSW government for a dedicated mother and baby unit in the northern New South Wales local health district and got in touch not long after. She needs 20,000 signatures.

> In NSW, there are currently two MBUs in Sydney, with an additional unit in development. These highly specialised units are not readily available within our community and while women from NNSW LHD are eligible for referral, the distance to travel and significant dislocation from the community and family support makes this service highly unattainable.

Melinda's little one is now sixteen months old and appears onscreen with a grin and a wave. As she recovered, Melinda found herself thinking of a woman she met in hospital whose daughter had been through something similar. Her outrage was growing.

'I know how bad I was, how much I was advocating for myself, and I still got to the point where I was twelve to twenty-four hours away from taking my own life. I was in disbelief that I was "enabled" or "allowed" to get that bad,' she says. 'I didn't want anyone else to suffer the systemic failure that I did. I was so broken, sick and out of it, but I was so determined when I was better to make sure people didn't fall through the same cracks I did.'

Melinda and I are similar in our desire for concrete action. She, too, believes that raising awareness and reducing stigma aren't enough. Yet advocacy for perinatal mental health for those in rural, regional and remote areas has been a lesson in understanding state and federal politics, the nature of funding and perseverance.

'It's been eye-opening to say the least,' Melinda says. 'I knew advocating in this space wasn't going to be easy and that I wouldn't be given everything on a silver platter. However, the political nature of advocacy has been very overwhelming at times. I constantly bring myself back to my core purpose of what I am doing and why.'

Over the past few months, Melinda has heard hundreds of stories of systemic failure and a lack of services, screening and perinatal expertise. 'Unfortunately, these stories don't trigger change,' she says. 'They absolutely do have their purpose and they are certainly powerful, but we need people power and the voices behind these stories to constantly push and drive change.'

Melinda's experience has changed the course of her life. 'Never ever would I have imagined this is what I would be doing,' she says of her advocacy. 'I thought I would have been back at work part-time while also being a mum. While my story and lived experience are the core of where I started, my advocacy role is no longer about *me* but about future mothers and families.'

Not long after I meet Melinda, I see a clip of NSW Greens MP Cate Faehrmann on Facebook. 'I note the minister's response today on the mother baby units, which I understand were opened today at the Royal Prince Alfred Hospital, as well as in Westmead and one other hospital,' she says in the video. 'That is wonder-ful, but the question was specifically about what the government is doing to assist rural, regional and remote New South Wales women who suffer what Melinda suffered. I urge the government to not wait for years before something is put in place.'

The news reports that a young mother has taken her own life, nine weeks after her baby was born. I read the article while in the car, collecting Hen from ballet. A reporter from News Ltd contacts my boss, Dr Nicole Highet, asking her for a comment.

On the radio, the announcer tells us that our suburb is going into lockdown again. It's the last day of the school term and around us, cases of Covid have been growing.

Just a few weeks earlier, I had sat with Nicole in a hotel room in Sydney, surrounded by printouts of our research data. We had highlighters in different colours for different themes – antenatal anxiety, depression, birth trauma, PTSD, psychosis, loneliness, the impact of Covid.

Almost 2000 expectant and new parents from around the country responded to our survey about the challenges faced from pre-conception through to the first year with a baby. The research, which is both qualitative and quantitative, will inform the basis of a national awareness campaign for which we've received Commonwealth funding.

I knew, of course, about the wounder healer, but I'd recently learnt of the 'vulnerable observer'. Anthropologist Ruth Behar argues that good qualitative research should 'break your heart'. Reading through the pages and pages of notes, I let my heart break.

There are stories of infertility, of multiple miscarriages and involuntary childlessness. Many women shared their experience of hyperemesis gravidarum (severe nausea and vomiting during pregnancy) and the brutal physical and emotional impacts of a condition still poorly understood by health professionals and the public. There are painful and at times harrowing accounts of birth trauma – experienced by not only women but also their partners.

Three men held me down while they ripped my daughter out of me.
I was treated like a statistic, not a mother.
My partner was traumatised too.

Many spoke of just how much their expectations about giving birth didn't match the reality, and how this left them feeling that they'd failed at motherhood before they'd even begun.

Despite doing four different antenatal classes, I felt completely unprepared for how traumatic it was.
I'll never be the same.

Some women shared that they'd felt dismissed or ignored by health professionals, that they weren't listened to, while others described being belittled.

Traumatic.
Upsetting.
Exhausting.
Unsettling.
Unfair.
Horrific.
Horrendous.
Disempowering.
Hell.

Many lamented the lack of continuity of care in the system, identifying that not having a familiar midwife only increased their anxiety and uncertainty during an already vulnerable time.

And while women shared that they'd been aware of postnatal depression, respondents said that other aspects of motherhood – such as antenatal depression and anxiety, loneliness, intrusive thoughts, postnatal rage, postnatal psychosis, PTSD and OCD – had taken them by surprise.

> *We need more education.*
> *I was completely unprepared.*
> *Why is there so much focus on the birth and nothing about what happens after?*
> *Everyone said, 'Oh well, at least you have a healthy baby.'*
> *No one tells you.*
> *No one tells you.*
> *No one tells you.*

The research, which took place during the prolonged Melbourne lockdown, also shows that Covid has taken an axe to the gaps in the system and made them deeper. We read stories of women going through their pregnancies with limited face-to-face antenatal care. Some went into labour without a support person. Many became parents while borders kept families around Australia apart, leaving them with limited social support or respite. Mothers' groups 'pivoted' to being online, making an already isolating time even more so.

For many expectant and new mothers, there is a profound sense of grief – for the experience of pregnancy or new motherhood that they'd longed for, coupled with anxiety about bringing a baby into a very different world.

In many areas, the research reiterates what we already know. And yet, it goes further in highlighting the stories behind the statistics we so often quote – and the barriers to seeking and receiving help.

We launch our subsequent campaign, The Truth, in March 2022. It aims to raise awareness of the *unique* and *broad range* of emotional and mental health challenges that many parents experience at each stage of the journey to parenthood and to educate health professionals, particularly around hyperemesis gravidarum, management of traumatic births, and the safe use of medication in pregnancy and while breastfeeding.

Informed by the findings of our research, we write and create short videos and information sheets on a range of topics, including postpartum rage, intrusive thoughts, shame and stigma, body image, birth trauma and, the one of which I'm most proud, postpartum psychosis. As part of our section on postpartum psychosis, Emily's dad also shared some of his experience of those 108 days Emily spent in psychiatric care. His words make me cry:

> Her mind was going at a million miles an hour nonstop talking, pacing around the room, talking to anyone (other patients) as if she could solve all their problems and still no sleep. I think it was about day three when we were told that Emily had been diagnosed with postpartum psychosis. My wife cried. I had no idea what this meant. The only positive news was that the doctors assured us that she would get better ... There is almost no teaching of mental illness in our school system, and the expectations on young mothers to be 'perfect' is quite unreasonable.
>
> We should be able to do better.

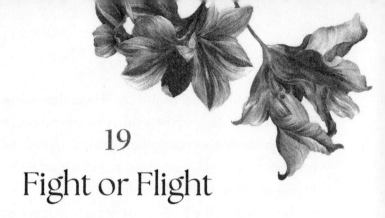

19

Fight or Flight

'If the illness in your brain is brutal,
be brutal back.'

ELIZABETH LYONS, *THE BLESSING OF DARK WATER*

The discharge summary from my time on the mother and baby unit arrives on a Friday afternoon. I've spent the day at the Multiple Birth Symposium in Parramatta, talking about COPE's research on the emotional and mental impacts of multiple births. I pour a glass of wine and open the envelope.

And the winner is …

Mood was pervasively ranging from 2–4/10. There had been moderate anhedonia [inability to feel pleasure] with diminished capacity to enjoy her infant. Appetite had been very poor with accompanying weight loss. There had been some suicidal thoughts without intent or plan over the past month. There had been no infanticidal ideation.

I'm still scanning the notes when Nicole calls to find out how the presentation went.

'It went well,' I tell her. 'And guess what? I got my records! From hospital. It says my postnatal risk questionnaire score was forty-two. What's the cut-off?'

'Twenty-three,' she says. 'Well, that's when you need to follow up.'

Always the overachiever.

After our call, I turn back to the summary.

On admission Ariane reported brittle mood and account suggesting sertraline had led to deterioration in her mental state. Of major concern to Ariane was the impact her illness was having on her relationship with Henry.

Mother-infant relationship difficulties subjectively described by Ariane.

Ariane began to experience fairly severe withdrawal effects including electric shock sensations. She received good feedback about Henry's attachment to her which was greatly reassuring.

There was some ambivalence around the benefit of group sessions – this was partly due to her professional status within the field.

There is genetic loading for mood disorder, perfectionistic traits may have been activated in the transition to motherhood. There was a long delay in seeking treatment likely because of the guilt and stigma associated with a mental health worker developing a mental illness.

Suggest graded return to work.

At the bottom of the form under follow-up agencies it says: *DoCS n/a.*

How strange it feels to see those words.

In my next session with Dr Q, I ask if we can talk about the discharge letter. I am at home, Zooming on the couch.

'Of course,' she says. 'What would you like to discuss?'

'Well, I'm interested in how different my scores are from admission to discharge,' I say. 'See the DASS depression score is twenty-eight and then on discharge it's four. I mean, it's clear that I just wanted to leave, right? Like I was just circling what I needed to in order to leave? Did they not realise I was fudging it? Did they really think their program was that good?'

Dr Q pauses in the way I've grown accustomed to. Over Zoom, with her face opposite mine, there's an almost visual gathering of her thoughts.

'I hear what you're saying,' Dr Q tells me. 'And I'm wondering how you feel about it.'

'About the scores?'

'Yeah.'

'Well, it's amusing, really.'

'No.' That pause again. 'That's a defence.'

'Is it?' I look out the window then back at the screen. 'No, I mean yes, you're right. It is. Alright, then … Maybe I'm a bit angry.'

'I think that might be right.'

'I think I'm angry no one said anything.'

'You were happy to be out, at the time, though,' Dr Q says. 'Remember?'

'Oh yes. I didn't want to be in there. I didn't think it was the right place for me at the time. But I am ten years older now. It just feels different, somehow.'

'They couldn't have made you stay.'

'That's true,' I say. 'They couldn't have.'

'It's okay to be angry about feeling like you slipped through the system, though. That's okay.'

'Yeah. I guess it is.' I pause. 'Dr Q?'

'Yes?'

'What does brittle mood mean? Is it a clinical term? It was in the summary.'

'Yes.' She laughs. 'Hmm … Unstable. Like a chocolate flake.'

'I thought it sounded poetic.'

'You think everything sounds poetic.'

⟳

I don't think I slipped through the cracks so much as skillfully avoided detection. Or is that the very same thing?

There are times, however, when the system can work – when planning and preparation, screening, treatment and the right care make a terrifying time slightly less so. But it's still far from perfect. This is Rebecca's story, which begins during her pregnancy and follows postpartum diagnoses of anxiety, fear of childbirth – known clinically as tokophobia – perinatal OCD and birth trauma. I met Rebecca online through her advocacy work and via her contribution to our national awareness campaign.

'I did postpartum planning,' Rebecca tells me over the phone. Her son has just started daycare, before she heads back to work after maternity leave. 'I was focused on postpartum depression, postpartum psychosis, postpartum anxiety.' But for Rebecca, this postpartum care planning became an obsession.

After undertaking prenatal screening with her obstetrician (in line with current guidelines to screen in early pregnancy), Rebecca was referred to a Gidget Foundation psychologist, as well as the social worker at the hospital where she was to deliver her first baby. She thought the anxiety would improve when her son arrived. What she didn't realise, and wouldn't for some months, was that her fixation on her postpartum mental health was a symptom of undiagnosed OCD.

As Rebecca's pregnancy progressed, her tokophobia also spiralled. 'The thought of birth was all consuming,' she says. 'I couldn't go any day or hour without thinking about it or worrying about it. The closer I got to birth, the more I felt I was taking one step closer to dying. I know a lot of people wouldn't understand that, but it felt so real.'

Now connected with the hospital social worker, Rebecca took a tour through the hospital and theatre in preparation for the birth. 'I have to credit my OB and this social worker,' she says. 'As unlucky as I got, I got very lucky with them.'

On paper, Rebecca's birth was 'textbook'. 'My social worker was allowed in the room,' she says. 'I think everyone knew how anxious I was, and they were all very beautiful. On paper I couldn't ask for a better team. But mentally and emotionally I was in fight-or-flight mode. Through the procedure I was having panic attack after panic attack. I couldn't feel my heart beating and that's usually what I rely on. *Am I alive? Is my heart going too fast? Let me breathe and regulate that.* But when you can't feel that, that thing you're relying on ...'

When staff asked Rebecca if she wanted to hold her son once the birth was over, her first response was 'no'. 'I was shaking,' she says. 'I just wanted to know, "How much longer will this take?" If I can just get through this birth, then it will be okay. If I just get through the thing that I'm scared of, I'll be okay. But that's not how it worked.'

The nightmares and other post-traumatic symptoms started two days later. 'All of a sudden, I had this rush of adrenaline. It felt like my body was on fire. I was back in fight-or-flight mode. My mind felt charged and wired. And from there I couldn't sleep.' Her fear of experiencing postpartum psychosis had also been an obsession during pregnancy, and it surfaced once again the more she tried to sleep. 'It became a fixation – another thing to be scared of,' Rebecca says. 'I remember saying in the hospital, "What if I get postpartum psychosis? I'm not sleeping. It's going to lead to psychosis." I thought I was going crazy.'

The social worker contacted a consultant psychiatrist, who on their second meeting told Rebecca, 'It's not the hormones, it's not the medication, it's clearly you. You've obviously idealised motherhood. Maybe you didn't want to be a mum. You didn't know what motherhood would really entail.' Those words would echo in her mind for months to come.

The medication prescribed for her anxiety made Rebecca feel numb and empty. So, now back at home, Rebecca turned to a local GP for help, telling them that the drugs were making her 'feel low'. 'There were no questions about OCD or intrusive thoughts,' she tells me. Instead, the GP assumed that the medication was causing her suicidal ideation.

But she wasn't suicidal. 'I remember saying, "I keep worrying that I'm going to hurt myself. But I don't want to hurt myself."That's why I was so distressed. No one said, "That's why you're performing compulsions." No one asked anything or even mentioned intrusive thoughts or mentioned they were normal during this period.'

Instead, the GP told her to present to emergency, where she would likely be sectioned and separated from her newborn. She chose to go home to her husband instead.

'The OCD, which I didn't know was OCD, took a nosedive,' Rebecca says. 'I was fixated on what if. What if I hurt myself? What if I hurt my son? Let me hide the scissors just in case I go crazy. Let me not look at the knives in the kitchen because what if I do something with them? It was that compulsive behaviour.'

Rebecca says she had harm OCD. 'I'm very anti-violent and the thought of hurting myself or someone else has always been a fear of mine. And it's always been there at the back of my mind, but it had never been at this acute place.'

To manage her fears, Rebecca would ask her husband to hold her for hours. 'I thought if I wasn't restrained then what if I'm capable of doing something?'

Desperate, Rebecca reached out to the social worker at the hospital, who arranged for her to be admitted to the MBU. Her son was just one week old. The same day, her breastmilk dried up.

On the MBU, Rebecca received diagnoses of OCD and PTSD. 'Once the distress had come down [and] the right medication had started to kick in, that's when I was able to pick up on the intrusive thoughts. I approached the psychiatrist and said, "I'm having this thought and I don't think I want to act on it, but it won't go away." She explained what ego-dystonic means – that it's against your values and that's why you're distressed by them. We did the OCD questionnaire and that's when we realised it had happened since I was a child.' Rebecca says the escalation of the OCD was a symptom of the PTSD. 'We were slowly chipping away [at what was going on] – insomnia, OCD, birth trauma. All of the symptoms made a lot more sense.'

Talking through Rebecca's experience, it's clear just how much the quality of antenatal and postnatal care depends on the individual clinicians. In Rebecca's case, although she was screened in line with best practice, referred to supports and given excellent antenatal care, an encounter with a psychiatrist who dismissed her symptoms and a GP who determined she was suicidal without further assessment only increased and prolonged her distress.

It's something she feels particularly passionate about now in her advocacy work. 'It's important that we're educating that first line of medical providers who you go and see because if they don't know, there's so much that can fall through the cracks,' she says. 'And they're the ones who are gatekeeping the mental health plans. A lot of us present to our GPs long before we present to emergency. Fortunately some are really brilliant – but there are others who want to wipe their hands clean of you and send you to ER.'

Since leaving hospital and celebrating her son's first birthday, Rebecca has started a podcast where she shares other women's stories of perinatal mental health. 'How much less alone would we feel if we just knew what others were going through?' she asks me. 'There shouldn't be stigma about going to a psych hospital or taking antidepressants. I wanted a space where we could tell our stories. Because that knowledge is power.'

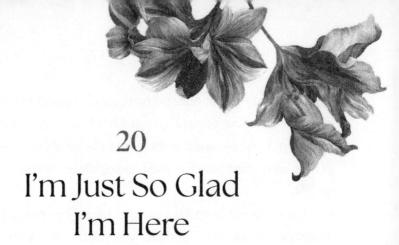

20

I'm Just So Glad
I'm Here

'Why bother?

*Because right now there is   someone
out there with
a wound   in the exact shape
of your words.'*

SEAN THOMAS DOUGHERTY

Henry and I are walking to the Sydney University book fair. It's a bright spring Saturday morning and he is giddy with excitement. The book fair is the first one after two years off during Covid and we've been looking forward to it all week. It's held in the Great Hall, next to the quadrangle where my parents were married almost fifty years ago.

'Do you only get one box?' Henry had asked me.

'Nah, mate,' I replied. 'You can have as many as you like.' (The boy is mine.)

We stop at the traffic lights on Parramatta Road and I check my phone. It's 10 September, World Suicide Prevention Day. *Shit,*

I think. It's been a busy week and I haven't scheduled a social media post for COPE. I open Google to search for an article on maternal suicide that I can pull some statistics from.

Suicide is one of the leading causes of maternal death …

'What are you doing, Mum?' Hen asks me, as we wait for the lights to change.

'Just looking for something for work,' I tell him.

'But we're going to the book fair,' he says. 'It's our *thing*.'

'Sorry, baby,' I say, putting my phone in my bag. 'Let's go.' The lights change and we cross the road, entering the gates of the uni. There are books to sift through and sausages to be eaten.

The post can wait.

Later, when I share the story with a friend who still works in child protection, he says, 'We need to have that worker self-care chat again. Why are you working on a Saturday?' He is half joking, though; he knows I can't stand the phrase self-care in the context of work and motherhood. I have a visceral reaction to the images it evokes: bubble baths, scented candles, sheet masks.

But I am learning boundaries. I am learning to read the limits of my own brain.

It's not easy. Recently, my friend Lauren sent me a meme on Instagram. It was a picture of two women, one with a sword through her neck. The text above it was, 'That friend that says they're fine even when they clearly aren't'.

'You,' Lauren wrote. 'You're literally on fire: "I'm good, but how are YOUUUUU."'

࿐

It's Perinatal Mental Health Week and I can feel myself sliding into a depressive episode. It is, perhaps, unsurprising – although it's the fifth year I've worked during it, it's the first I've managed while writing a memoir about the same subject.

My thoughts feel fuzzy around the edges. Unformed. I confuse the names of students in my adult ballet class, something I never do. I am exhausted even though I'm sleeping well. I hear Dr Q's words reverberating in my head: *We have to protect your sleep.* I have been working too much, too hard – teaching toddler ballet, working on COPE's new psychoeducation app, presenting at conferences and writing this book.

We don't often talk about the aftermath of a breakdown, the kind that has changed the fabric of who you are, what you're made of. People want a neat story: I was unwell and I recovered. But it's never that simple. Even after you're better and no longer just living but thriving, if you've lost your mind once before, you carry the fear of losing it again.

It's strange, this constant looking behind and looking ahead, this learning to live in the space between. Is a trick of the light just that – the light playing tricks? Or is my mind losing its grasp? Yes, this time, it's just tricky light. Breathe out, breathe in – you're not seeing things. Not this time.

I read a paper on the experiences of women who suffered from postnatal psychosis and how they made sense of their lives afterwards. I'm not the only one who second-guesses my senses. 'Women felt that the illness took away the ability to experience normal emotions,' the authors note. Like me, these mums often worried that high or low moods might be reflective of another mental health episode rather than the normal variations of life.

'Are you crashing?' Robb will ask if I'm starting to slow down, if he finds keys in the fridge or milk in the cupboard with the coffee cups. 'You have that look in your eye.' He tries to hide it, but there's often fear in his voice. 'A bit elevated?' he'll enquire if I'm talking too fast, more agitated than usual or deep-cleaning the house at eleven p.m.

I am aware now of the signs, of what I need to do when my brain feels full of holes or leaps ahead too fast for me to catch. I make an appointment with Dr Q. I dance until my limbs are sore. I go to bed early, read poems, text my friends and rest and rest and rest.

Martha Graham once said, 'To me the body says what words cannot.' When I am anxious, I dance until I'm breathless. All I need is an empty studio or a balcony and a piece of music. When the anxiety vibrates, I move to discharge it – purging it through my sweat and limbs and the shapes my body makes – big and small and ephemeral.

Not long after lockdown ended, my friend texted, 'One time in a message, maybe a month ago, you weren't doing so well, and you told me you were just focusing on making small shapes. And I thought that was such a cute and poetic typo, and because you weren't so well, I didn't ask what you actually meant. A month later I've realised it wasn't a typo. My friend was helping me put my arm in the right place (up in 5th?) and she said that ballet is all shapes and lines. You were making small shapes. And I get it. When I'm struggling, tired, over-stimulated, or just need to withdraw, my voice is small. My handwriting is small. My body feels physically so tiny. So dancing is making shapes in time, and sometimes we need to make small ones. And slow ones.'

⁀

'Hidden pain, controlled bodies: does ballet have to be like this?' I am on the floor in the studio, waiting for my adult dancers to arrive, when this *Jezebel* headline comes into my feed. I manoeuvre myself into a lazy middle split and lean forwards on my elbows to read, smirking at the irony. It's how I used to study all those years ago in high school, doing my homework on the ground while stretching or doing pilates – always twisting, contorting, strengthening.

The article quotes former ballet dancer and writer Sophie Charles:

> We were systematically lied to since childhood that the skills that we acquired in the ballet world would serve us in our next endeavour, and for me, it was the opposite. I tried applying what worked for me in the ballet world to being a mother for the first time, and it was completely catastrophic. My perfectionism, my determination, my hard work, my self-sacrifice … all the things that make a great dancer completely wrecked me mentally and physically as a mother …
>
> It becomes necessary in ballet to hide your inner life so your outside can seem serene. I was able to do that for the first seven months of new motherhood while I was miserable and suffering on the inside: I didn't ask for help and just continued pushing myself to the brink. The internal monologue during ballet was often, 'Well, I survived this, I made it through' … literally life or death talk. And that's the level that I would push myself oftentimes with postpartum depression. I almost didn't make it. I almost didn't survive.

I love ballet, but gosh, it really did a number on me.

⤳

When I start writing this book, I make an appointment to see a new GP, while Dr Q is on extended leave over the winter. 'I feel blunted,' I tell him, walking through my history and the medication I still take each night – the SSRI, the mood stabiliser and the antipsychotic for sleep. 'I feel as though I can't access any emotions. I know cognitively what the emotion should feel like, and I know the behaviour and actions I should take in response, but it's as though the actual emotion is blocked off to me. I just think, maybe I'd like to be able to feel while I'm writing this book.'

The GP laughs. 'I can understand that.' He opens my file. 'Alright, then. Let's try to find you a feeling.'

Together, we decide to cut down my dosage of Lexapro, the antidepressant I've taken for nine years. 'It's something I hear often,' the GP explains as he prints off a script for my new dosage. 'The blunting. It can be difficult to get the balance right, so let's just take it slowly and see how you go.'

He's right. It takes about six weeks, but on a lower dose life rushes back in a way I've not felt in years. I feel sadness again, and the pain of digging through these memories, lifting them out, inspecting them, deciding which ones to follow. But there's joy, too – a spontaneity, a vitality.

One review of the evidence describes emotional blunting as 'a sense of numbing of both positive and negative emotions'. 'Patients who suffer from emotional blunting are subject to a reduction in a broader range of emotions, including love, affection, fear and anger.' Is it a side effect of medication or a residual aspect of major depression? Studies are mixed and the jury is still out. Neuropsychological implications aside, what does it mean for the self to be let loose after being bound in cotton-wool? I am excited to find out who I am again with less padding.

My decision to taper comes at the same time as the debate around antidepressant use rages once again. An article in *Nature* challenges the idea that depression is caused by a chemical imbalance in the brain, particularly serotonin. 'We suggest it is time to acknowledge that the serotonin theory of depression is not empirically substantiated,' the authors write. But, as the research hits the news cycle, experts around the world urge caution: don't stop taking your medication without speaking to your doctor, and for god's sake don't go cold turkey.

I am reminded, as I was when I was a patient in hospital, just how much we still don't know.

～

A woman I met in a peer support group is now in the new Naamuru Parent and Baby Unit at Royal Prince Alfred Hospital in Sydney. Naamuru, which means leading the way, opened in May 2022 and is NSW's first public MBU. During the school holidays, Hen and I are walking past the clinic when I tell him that I want to drop something into her. I've visited the new facility a few times now and am delighted to see how well designed and welcoming it is.

'My friend is in the hospital,' I tell him. 'How about you head home? I won't be long behind you.'

'Is she sick?' he asks.

'She just had a baby,' I say. 'And she needs some help with her mental health.'

'Oh, right,' he says. 'Like anxiety?'

'Exactly. Like anxiety.' I pause as we walk down King Street towards the clinic. 'I needed some help too, you know. When you were about nine months old. I got really sick. We stayed in a similar place. This one is much nicer and newer. But that's where I met Carolyn and Jackson.'

'Really?'

'Yeah. You know that video I've showed you where you're pushing the baby walker up and down the hallways?'

'I pushed it into the wall.'

I laugh. 'Yes, that one. That was in the hospital. You stayed with me there for a little while.'

'Can I come and have a look?' The question takes me by surprise.

'If you want to, sure. I'll just text her to make sure it's okay.'

'Of course!' she replies. 'See you soon!'

Inside, my friend smiles and waves us both in. She looks healthier than when I saw her last, the colour returning to her cheeks. We walk down the corridor of the ward and head outside into the sun where there's play equipment.

'This is *my* baby,' I tell my friend, giving Hen a kiss on the cheek. I hand her a picture book I bought for her daughter. 'We were exactly where you are,' I say. 'Exactly.'

And look at us now, baby. Look at us now.

∽

Dr Q and I have our eleventh anniversary as I'm writing this chapter. 'Second-longest relationship of my life,' I tell her.

Not long after, I read an article Andrew Solomon wrote after the death of his therapist.

Late in our work, I said that I was in chaotic depression and felt like I was melting away. He looked at me for a minute, then said, 'If you turn into a pool of water, I'll find a glass.' Some people go into therapy because they want to be released from their constraints. I wanted to break out of some of mine, and I did – but what I really wanted was containment. When I discovered and achieved ways to break free, he consistently found the glass.

My feet are so firmly planted here – in life and love and work and words and dance – that it's hard to believe I had to fight so hard to stay alive.

Let me hold onto the hope for you, Dr Q once said. And she did – still does – keep finding the glass.

I send Dr Q a podcast episode in which Nicole interviews me for the Mental Health Professionals' Network. I had mentioned it during one of our sessions and she texts me after to remind me to send it to her. I feel like a preschooler showing her my finger-painting, hoping she'll like it enough to put it up on the fridge. Those signs of transference are everywhere.

'Did you listen to it?' I ask during our next session.

'Of course.'

'What did you think?'

'I think you sounded excellent. I learnt things you'd never told me.'

'Yeah?'

'Yeah.' That pause again. 'However … I think when you were talking about me, you put a little Vaseline on the lens there, dear.'

But there's a smile on her lips.

⸎

Mum tells anyone who will listen that I am writing a book about perinatal mental health – her hairdresser, her students, her bank tellers.

'The number of times I've spoken to women recently and they've said they suffered in silence,' she texts me. 'But it's so good it's being taken seriously.'

Her words make me teary. That she is flying the flag, that she is sending out ripples of awareness far and wide, means more than she will ever know.

Everyone keeps asking me if writing this book is cathartic. I know they want my answer to be yes – but the truth is, it isn't cathartic, not really. I can't cry, so I don't, but I tear at my skin like I used to when I was a child. I drink too much wine, shrink inwards away from friends and family. I wake myself up calling out in my sleep. I answer the DoCS helpline in my dreams. I lose my appetite, watch my hip bones sharpen.

I think of Annie Ernaux, who says that what counts is not the things that happen but what we do with them. And I keep writing.

Where do I put it down?

I come across a piece by the writer Erin Vincent, whose memoir about the death of her parents I read recently. 'About a year into the writing I wondered why I was so tired all the time; why after writing for an hour or two all I would want to do was sleep,' she says in *The Guardian*. 'I thought I was just being lazy, so I pushed myself harder.' In fact, Vincent pushed herself to the brink of suicide. In her essay, Vincent cites the work of Dr Bessel van der Kolk, who says that 'flashbacks and reliving are in some ways worse than the trauma itself' because while a traumatic experience 'has a beginning and an end', a flashback can happen anywhere and for any length of time.

Vincent describes the process of dredging up the past and writing about it as 'self-inflicted torture'. But it's not just difficult for me – it's not easy for Robb, either. I am constantly probing his memories, testing my recollections against his. I know he wants the writing to be over soon, for me to come back again. I know he worries about the impact it's having on my head. But I also know he understands how much I need to get it all down – and why. At first, I wanted to share my story. Then I wanted to understand it. Now, I need it to help herald change.

I feel so very loved, so very cared for.

'I am almost there,' I tell him.

⌇

'I wish you'd asked for help.'

'I'm sorry I was so far away.'

'I had no idea.'

'You looked so happy on social media.'

I feel so much guilt for not speaking up.

I carry the guilt of my loved ones who simply didn't know.

It is no one's fault.

If I've learnt anything about being unwell during the perinatal period, it's the need for help to reach IN, rather than waiting for new parents to reach out. So often, they simply won't. Instead of saying, 'Let me know if there's anything I can do,' be the friend or relative who takes an older sibling to the park while mum is adjusting to the shock of having two. Drop over a meal or pay for a cleaner. Ask new parents how they are and be prepared to listen, to rally support if they need it. I may not have called the PANDA helpline when Brooke texted it to me, but I'll never forget that she took the time to look it up and share it with me. She listened, she cared, and she trusted her instincts. It also gently planted the seed that maybe, perhaps, could it be that I wasn't really okay?

Listen to the silences. If a friend stops replying to messages or starts to withdraw, I'd urge you to keep checking in. Gently. They may not feel like they're able to respond, but they won't forget that you're there and that you're not giving up on them.

There's a phrase I see on Instagram along the lines of, 'Don't just hold the baby, hold the mum.' I think about what it means to be held and contained – to be anchored to time and space in those early, blurry months when neither seem to make sense.

'*Holding on for dear life*', Karen Kleiman writes. 'That's how one woman explained it. It's the perfect description of what postpartum women in despair describe. *It feels like I will never get better. I will go crazy. I will die.*'

✍

While writing the final words of this book, I see a post on Instagram from Ireland Baldwin, daughter of Alec Baldwin and Kim Bassinger. It's now common to see celebrities share their experiences of pregnancy and postpartum mental illness, but it's often done years after the fact – neat, processed and pithy. But Ireland is in the thick of it – and it's difficult to read.

> Vulnerability trigger warning. I'm not writing this post for sympathy. I'm only posting this because I personally have found comfort in unfamiliar corners of social media during this time in my life. Social media is very toxic and misleading, but I have found community in times where I felt no one understands. I'm sharing my innermost feelings with the hope that someone will read this and feel less alone. I came across various posts and videos where people were just fucking honest about how hard this journey can be and it's helped me so much.

Baldwin is right: social media can be a wild and overwhelming place for expectant and new mothers. And yet it remains one of the few ways they can stay connected while isolated at home with a newborn. A middle ground between the wilderness and the camaraderie is often hard to find. Curating COPE's feed, I struggle with the toxic positivity I see on Instagram, the pastel Canva tiles with 'You got this mama!' or 'Tiger stripes are sexy' or 'Enjoy every minute, you only get 18 summers'. (What the shit is that last one about?)

When you haven't 'got this' and when you're struggling with complicated feelings around your postpartum body and mind, it's unhelpful and condescending to be told what to feel. And while I love the concept of matrescence and the way it explains the profound changes in all aspects of a new mother's life, I don't love the way it's been commodified by some. On social media, matrescence coaches, matrescence guides and matrescence educators (all with varying degrees of qualifications and expertise) seem to be trying to capitalise on this word du jour. There's even a wellness brand, Matrescence Skin, which claims, 'The journey to motherhood can be complicated, but your skincare routine doesn't have to be.' Did you know you can trademark an academic term? I didn't – but there you go.

I often hear from women who blame themselves for struggling with something so 'natural'. They diligently take their medication, go to therapy, practise 'self-care' and, like I did, wonder why they don't get better and how they've managed to 'fail' at recovery, too.

In 1980, sociologist Ann Oakley released her book *Women Confined*, in which she argued that society is a major instigator of postpartum depression. Reviewing the book, *Time* magazine writes, 'The recipe for the depression is to create an unrealistic myth about motherhood, offer unfeeling medical care, and then set the new mother down in a social system that offers her little support for her new child and new role.'

It's a sentiment captured forty years later in this viral tweet by Ramblin Mama:

> Moms: We are drowning. Help.
> Everyone: Wow you're superhuman!
> Moms: What? No. Can you just hel—
> Everyone: I don't know how you do it!
> Moms: We're not. Help us.
> Everyone: OMG you're amazing tho

And there's the rub: screening, prevention and treatment will never be the full story when it comes to combating perinatal mental illness. We can't ignore the social and political context in which we mother, in which we parent.

Eliane Glaser writes, 'Mothers are trying too hard, and society is not trying nearly hard enough.' But, she says, big improvements are within reach. 'Proper care before, during and after birth; a rethink of work for both women and men, and the transformation of society's incessant chastising of mothers into due value and respect. Motherhood is feminism's unfinished business.'

She is right, and her book *Motherhood: A Manifesto* is not so much a rallying cry but a roar. However, white feminism isn't enough. There's precious little written about intersectional feminism and perinatal mental health. I do find a paper published in 2018 in which Natalie Stevens and her colleagues look at the effectiveness of a coordinated perinatal mental healthcare model in the US, using an intersectional feminist perspective. Of the model itself, the authors note that it was developed:

... with an appreciation of the perinatal period as a time of profound physical, psychological, and social transition, and that each woman's experience of the challenges associated with this transition are shaped by myriad intersecting social factors. Using an intersectional perspective, perinatal women's vulnerability is characterized in terms of power versus oppression; in other words, to what degree does a woman enjoy numerous material benefits versus face racial discrimination and traumatic stress in order to meet her and her family's most basic material needs? Or, to what extent does her social environment support her perinatal mental wellbeing or actively undermine it?'

But while the researchers describe the findings as promising, they note that disparities remain an enormous public health concern that need to be addressed. This is, of course, true of services in Australia, too.

I am thinking of the writers I turned to, to understand this transition, to understand matrescence: a word I didn't know existed. There's Winnicott, of course, who not only brought us the idea of the good-enough mother but, in a seminal essay in the 1940s, wrote a long list of reasons a mother might 'hate' her baby.

The baby is a danger to her body in pregnancy and at birth. He tries to hurt her, periodically, bites her all in love. He is suspicious, refuses her good food, and makes her doubt herself, but eats well with his aunt. After an awful morning with him she goes out and he smiles at a stranger who says, 'Isn't he sweet!'

270

I am thinking of Adrienne Rich, whose book *Of Woman Born* was recommended to me by a mentor from my child protection days. Her description of the push and pull and pain and love and mess and magic of motherhood is perhaps unparalleled. 'My children cause me the most exquisite suffering of which I have any experience,' Rich writes. 'It is the suffering of ambivalence: the murderous alternation between bitter resentment and raw-edged nerves, and blissful gratification and tenderness and intolerance.'

Gratification, tenderness, intolerance.

I am thinking of Rachel Cusk: 'I remain fascinated by where you go once you are a mother. And if you ever come back.'

I am thinking of something I wrote on my notes app at some point while writing this book, a midnight thought that makes no sense upon waking: *I am all the mothers I have ever been.* I don't know what I meant but, sitting here now, I am thinking about the mothers I've been and am and will be. I am thinking of all these versions of myself: the one who watched the two lines appear on the pregnancy test; the one who walked through pregnancy wrapped in anxiety she couldn't and wouldn't name; the one who slowly, painfully, brutally lost her mind postpartum; the one who, when she finally recovered, adores being a mother to the most wonderful, clever, kind boy.

I did go, but I have returned.

∽

'What did it look like when I started to come back?' I ask Robb. We are out for dinner, sitting opposite one another in a restaurant.

'Your smile was genuine,' he says. 'You would show genuine joy. Leaving the house to do things – going back into society. You'd go to the bookshop, to Gould's, and you'd come back with all these books we didn't have room for. But you were going somewhere! You were back to doing things with purpose. And that day you pulled your pointe shoes on in your parents' kitchen. There's that photo I took, and you had a big beaming smile. It was just you – discovering you again.'

I learn on TikTok that flamingos lose their pink colouring while raising their chicks because they give them so much of their food and energy. At some point, though, it comes back. That's how I feel – like I've finally got my pink back.

Writing has helped with this too. And then one day, a day I never really thought would come, Henry is hovering at the end of the printer in Officeworks, ready to catch the first draft of my book. He is so proud of me that my heart is doing somersaults.

'Are we crowning?' I ask, as the printer fires up.

'Are we what?' Hen asks.

There were times when writing this book felt a little like pregnancy. I am not the first to make this comparison, I know, and yet I was surprised by how physical it felt. 'I want it out of me,' I once joked to a friend. 'I am carrying it around and it is taking up space inside of me. I want it out.'

When all the pages have been printed (Mum and bub doing well), Hen and Robb disappear conspiratorially, leaving me staring at the traffic on Parramatta Road. I feel a newborn-like exhaustion, but there's excitement underneath it, too.

Ten minutes later they emerge and Henry hands me my book; my boys have had it bound for me.

And I am tired and elated and the balloon that is not being able to cry expands and expands and expands until it pops and the tears come.

But they are happy tears.

⟋⟍

This is what I've learnt about recovery from perinatal mental illness.

You are not a burden – not to your friends or your family or your child. They're not better off without you. Let me say that again: they are not better off without you.

We all have moments in our lives when we need to rely on and ask for help from others; it's simply your turn. Asking for support when you need it, and accepting it when it's offered, is one of the bravest things you can do. In my experience, and in the experience of so many others, people want to help. They just don't know how. Let them in.

Getting better isn't linear. There will be days when you will feel as though someone has picked you up from a hard-fought point in your recovery and thrown you backwards. The tears will be close to the surface; your heart will hurt. But you won't have fallen as far as it feels, and it will be just that little bit easier to get back up.

If you feel as though you've lost your hope, let others carry it for you. Let your family and your friends and your doctor, psychologist, psychiatrist (or whichever professional you're engaged with) hold it for safekeeping. Let them believe that you'll get well. Eventually, you'll believe it too.

At times, you'll wonder when you'll start to feel like yourself again. And the truth is that you won't. Not completely, anyway. You can't help but come through to the other side of perinatal mental illness – or motherhood, really – changed. You'll see the world differently. It's hard to explain, because it will vary for everyone, but I hope you'll find there's a richness to life, an appreciation of the simple pleasures and a knowledge of the rhythm of sadness. And that this knowledge and appreciation builds resilience and a steely inner strength you'll draw on for years to come.

At some point, as you start to feel better, you'll realise just how unwell you have been. With the clarity of recovery comes a deep and incredibly painful awareness of the time you've lost. The grief may take you by surprise. But the sadness will lessen gradually as you seize the present – and as you look to the future with hope and health.

You will fall in love with life again. It will happen slowly and then, one day, you'll be dancing with your little one in the lounge room, or swimming in the ocean, or tasting coffee – actually tasting it instead of gulping it down – and you'll smile and know that you're getting there.

And you will get there. Let me hold that hope for you.

Epilogue

It's RUOK? Day and Hen is listening to me talk about a post I need to write for COPE. He is eating breakfast when he turns to me with a grin. 'You good, Brah?' he says.

'Brah?' I laugh. 'Brah?'

Who knew the transition from Mummy to Mum to Brah would happen so quickly.

I am, though, my darling. I am okay. In fact, I am better than okay. And you, Hen, are the best thing I've ever done.

Appendix

Awareness of perinatal mental health conditions
For decades, the primary focus of perinatal mental health has been on postnatal depression. Yet it is just one of many conditions that women (and fathers and partners) experience during pregnancy and the postnatal period. There is less public awareness about depression and anxiety during pregnancy, birth trauma, psychosis and perinatal OCD.

Research conducted by PANDA in 2016, building on Nicole Highet's work at Beyond Blue, found that 52 per cent of Australians identified depression as a key health issue after having a baby – an increase from 45 per cent in 2009. However, only 5 per cent identified depression or anxiety as a key health issue during pregnancy. Additionally, 60 per cent of the community didn't realise men can experience perinatal anxiety and depression.

A study by Gidget Foundation Australia in 2023 noted that 55 per cent of new parents don't know how to spot the signs of perinatal anxiety and depression. This is particularly true for postnatal psychosis. When I ask the women in the Beyond Postnatal Psychosis Facebook group if anyone had heard of the illness prior to their diagnosis, not one said they had. One shared that it had come up in her Google searches when she knew something wasn't right, 'at god knows what time of the morning', but that she had skimmed over it because of how rare it was. Another told me that despite working in mental health, she too had never heard of postpartum psychosis.

My aim is not to scare women and their families. But being able to identify postpartum psychosis – whether in a partner, a friend, a colleague or relative – can, quite literally, save lives.

Three years ago, a US team led by Kristina Dulaney created the first Perinatal Psychosis Awareness Day, which takes place annually on 5 May. This year, I joined a group of women who host gatherings in different time zones around the world for those who've experienced postpartum psychosis. We laughed, we cried, and we talked about the different resources and services available in our parts of the globe. Through these gatherings, I also met men who've lost their wives to perinatal mental illness, and I learned of the advocacy and fundraising work they're doing in their beloveds' names. How do you go on? The work these men are doing is critical and brutal.

Celebrities are starting to speak up now, too. 'I had 22 hours of postpartum psychosis on day three,' singer/songwriter Paloma Faith said publicly after her own psychotic break in 2021. It's the first time I've heard someone high-profile speak about the condition. 'I was so tired that I completely lost track of what was going on. I was having a hallucination. I thought they'd sewn my head to the body of someone else … I was crying and asking, "What have you done to me?" when I pressed the nurse button.'

Australian actress Sarah Wynter wrote about her harrowing experience with postpartum psychosis for *Vanity Fair* in January 2022:

> Maybe I was playing a part. I'd never been a Method actor, but maybe I was in a movie playing someone with a brain injury. Maybe I had delved so deeply into my character that I couldn't

let go. There was an audience and a director somewhere—*Please show yourself, director!* Where was the rest of the cast? What was real? Did I have twin babies, or was that my character? I didn't know who I was.

She also spoke about it on *60 Minutes*, noting that it had taken her over a decade to publicly talk about her experience due to stigma and shame. 'I'm just trying to de-stigmatise mental illness, maternal mental health and the act of asking for help.'

Hearing about postpartum psychosis in the absence of tragedy is crucial. As I write this chapter, there are multiple news reports of maternal suicide and infanticide here and overseas. Although many note that the mother was experiencing postpartum depression, we know from the research that psychosis is often missed.

These stories are often reported under the guise of raising awareness, yet serve only to reinforce stigma or perpetuate the myth that a depressed mum wants to kill or her hurt her child. Awareness-raising is important, and we know tragedies get clicks. But it can't be at the expense of ensuring that women feel safe to speak up about how they're feeling.

We don't have this balance right yet.

The cost of perinatal depression and anxiety

Of the approximately 600,000 parents who welcome a baby in Australia each year, about 60,000 mothers and 30,000 fathers will experience perinatal anxiety and depression. This affects around 61,000 children (accounting for multiple births). The impacts of this are not only mental and emotional, but also financial. A 2019 report by PricewaterhouseCoopers notes that perinatal depression and anxiety costs Australia $877 million annually. This is a conservative estimate, however, given that many studies have focused only on maternal postnatal depression and that other research gaps exist, particularly around Aboriginal and Torres Strait Islander parents, LGBTQI+ couples and those from culturally and linguistically diverse backgrounds.

Aboriginal and Torres Strait Islander parents
A study of maternity patients at the Royal Women's Hospital in Melbourne, published in *BMC Pregnancy and Childbirth* in 2018, found that Aboriginal and Torres Strait Islander mothers were more likely to have been diagnosed with a mental illness (49.5 per cent) than non-Indigenous mothers (18.8 per cent). As part of the National Postnatal Depression Research Program – where 40,000 women in Australia were screened – 19 per cent of Indigenous women had antenatal depression, compared with 8.9 per cent of non-Indigenous women. Postnatally, 12 per cent had depression, compared with 7.6 per cent of non-Indigenous women. Additionally, 6.3 per cent had both antenatal and postpartum depression, compared with 2.7 per cent of non-Indigenous women.

But our system continues to fail and to punish Indigenous parents – many of whom face the continuing intergenerational impacts of the Stolen Generations. 'Perinatal services now have more trained experts than ever,' note the authors of the 2022 paper *Supporting Aboriginal and Torres Strait Islander Families to Stay Together from the Start (SAFeST Start)*. 'Yet, parents experiencing social and emotional complexity are often referred from the therapeutic health sector to the CPS statutory sector for "support".' As the authors highlight, antenatal care isn't considered safe by many Aboriginal and Torres Strait Islander parents, in part out of fear that their baby will be removed. Yet avoiding antenatal care also often triggers risk-of-harm notifications. During 2019–2020, one in five Indigenous children admitted into out-of-home care were less than twelve months old. As Cath Chamberlain and her colleagues note, 'These figures represent compounding intergenerational trauma and institutional harm to Aboriginal and Torres Strait Islander families and communities.'

According to the *Family Matters* report, published in November 2023, the number of Aboriginal and Torres Strait Islander children affected by the child protection system is increasing. As the authors note, 'In 2022 there were 22,328 Aboriginal and Torres Strait Islander children in out-of-home care in Australia, the highest number ever recorded. Most disturbingly, Aboriginal and Torres Strait Islander children are 10.5 times more likely than non-Indigenous children to be in out-of-home care.'

We know, too, that when babies are removed at or after birth, parents rarely receive acceptable and effective support, despite risk-of-harm notifications prior to the birth. As outlined in the NSW government's *Family Is Culture* report:

> Newborn removals are highly traumatic for the birth parents, with birth mothers recounting feelings of shock, pain, sorrow, disbelief, anxiety, guilt, shame and emptiness upon the removal of their babies. Birth mothers and fathers are left to live in an 'in-between state where their child is gone but did not die', and the complexity and depth of their grief can lead to serious and longstanding psychological damage. This may then have a significantly detrimental effect on their later experiences of pregnancy and parenthood. It is widely recognised in the literature relating to compulsory child removals that many women suffer 'a downturn in functioning' post removal. Anecdotal evidence indicates that women may 'seek comfort in a further pregnancy'. This may lead to successive removals of newborns from the woman's care.

In a 2014 national survey by COPE, 98 per cent of providers of perinatal care identified trauma, stress and grief as significantly affecting Aboriginal and Torres Strait Islander mothers, yet almost half (43 per cent) did not feel satisfied their service could address these issues.

There's also research showing that Western approaches are inappropriate for the needs of Indigenous families. The EPDS, for example, hasn't been validated for use with Indigenous parents. Work is occurring in this space with the *Baby Coming You Ready?* digital platform and the Kimberley Mum's Mood Scale, which adapts the EPDS to incorporate discussion or yarning about psychosocial risk and protective factors.

But there's always more work to be done.

Universal screening for perinatal depression and anxiety
Australia's clinical guidelines recommend that women are screened for depression and anxiety twice during pregnancy (as early as possible and again at around twenty-eight weeks) and twice in the year after having a baby. We know, however, that in practice who is screened and when varies. Research shows, for example, that women who give birth in the public health system are more likely to be assessed across all psychosocial domains than women in the private system.

While the absence of a national approach to data collection has made it difficult to assess trends, the introduction of digital screening is changing that. A 2020 study, which relied on self-reports, found that one in five women are not screened both antenatally and postnatally. Mums who reported emotional distress prior to birth were less likely to have been screened both during pregnancy and after the birth. As the authors highlight, this is concerning given we know previous mental health issues are one of the strongest risk factors for perinatal depression.

As well as screening for symptoms of depression and anxiety, the national guidelines recommend that psychosocial factors are explored. The postnatal risk questionnaire (PNRQ) and its pregnancy equivalent (the ANRQ, developed in Australia) look at psychosocial aspects that may place a woman at higher risk of experiencing a perinatal mental health issue, including a history of mental health issues; the presence of any major stressors such as bereavement, job loss or relationship breakdown; degree of practical and emotional support; history of physical, sexual or emotional abuse; levels of perfectionism and anxiety. (The PNRQ is the measure on which I received excellent marks in the MBU.) In its more recent form, the ANRQ also screens for substance abuse and family violence.

COPE received Commonwealth funding to roll-out iCOPE, a digital screening platform, in all Maternal, Child and Family Health Centres and public maternity hospitals. iCOPE includes the EPDS and the psychosocial risk measures – and is available in twenty-five different languages. We will soon have audio versions available too, removing more barriers to screening. Implementation across the states and territories, however, has been slow. At the time of writing, only Victoria has started using iCOPE, although South Australia, Queensland and the Northern Territory have all signed up. Early evaluation of data in Victoria has shown not only that rates of screening have increased, but also that screening rates of those from non-English speaking backgrounds have increased too.

Screening for psychosis is more complex. Unlike perinatal depression and anxiety, there are no screening tools specifically designed for postpartum psychosis. But that doesn't mean we can't screen for it. We can ask about established risk factors, including personal or family history of bipolar disorder as well as previous episodes of psychosis after childbirth, remembering that these may not always have been diagnosed. Health professionals who see women in the immediate postpartum period, before the six-week check-up, should also be alert for symptoms.

Referral pathways and expert treatment
Screening is only effective if referral pathways are available for those identified as at risk or needing further support, as are clinicians with expertise in perinatal mental health.

After a review in 2022 of the Better Access program, federal health minister Mark Butler announced that Medicare-rebatable psychology sessions would be reduced from twenty to ten from 1 January 2023. How is this likely to affect perinatal mental health care? We know that clients often require more than one appointment per month, particularly in the acute stages of perinatal ill-health.

Treating postpartum women is not straightforward – and nor should we expect it to be.

Discovering Karen Kleiman's work was a revelation. So much of my own experience of being a patient made sense when I read her book *Therapy and the Postpartum Woman*. I thought numerous times while writing this book, *Why didn't you just ask for help? Why were you such a difficult patient?* But Kleiman's clinical experience validates my own lived experience. 'Most women with new babies are not interested in psychotherapy,' Kleiman writes. 'This is not to say that they are unwilling to engage in the process of healing. It means it does not make sense or fit into their world right now and they simply have no time for it.' Kleiman says that although therapists without perinatal expertise can be effective, 'women who receive help from therapists who have received specialized training, who have cultivated a deeper understanding of the impact postpartum depression and anxiety can have on a family, who have developed the skills to connect with the gravity of postpartum complexities, well, they get better, *better*'.

This type of work can be difficult, as Professor Anne Buist knows. 'It's hard to sit with the patient, to reparent them or to help them reflect. It's time-consuming,' she says. 'You have to sit with them getting worse. Sit with them hating you. That takes a particular personality style.'

Professor Buist has found that group therapy can be particularly effective. She tells me about a twenty-week outpatient program she ran with women who'd had a previous hospital admission and had CBT therapy. In groups, they recorded then watched themselves doing the Strange Situation scenario with their babies. 'It was like psychotherapy on speed,' she says. All the women learned from discussing one another's videos. 'We'd say, "I wonder what the baby needs here?" And they'd come up with it themselves. And that's where the power of change came from. Some of them still needed an individual therapist to go on with afterwards to resolve their issues with their parents. But they were able to put their issues aside and bond with their baby and stop intergenerational transmission happening. It was extraordinary.'

Mother and Baby Units

It's well established that keeping mums and babies together for treatment is best practice, as recommended in the National Clinical Guidelines and by the Royal Australian and New Zealand College of Psychiatrists. But there simply aren't enough units or beds.

Until early 2022, New South Wales had no public beds at all. Before then, St John of God in Burwood, a private hospital, was the only option for new mothers needing in-patient support.

A second eight-bed unit for the state was announced in September 2021 and opened in 2023. It's good news but it's difficult to fathom why it's taken so long.

Victoria has six units, Perth has two, while South Australia and Queensland have one each. There are currently no public units in Tasmania, the Northern Territory or the ACT, which means that if a mother requires urgent care and doesn't have private health insurance, she will be admitted to a general unit – without her baby.

According to the UK Royal College of Psychiatrists, one eight-bed unit is needed for every 15,000 deliveries. In 2021 the Australian Bureau of Statistics recorded 309,996 births. New South Wales had the most with 99,300, followed by Victoria with 76,414, Queensland with 64,261, Western Australia with 34,065, South Australia with 19,783, the ACT with 6410, Tasmania with 6027 and the Northern Territory with 3736.

Based on these figures, Australia should have about 168 beds in around 21 units. Instead, we have 83 beds across 13 units. Only Victoria meets the UK's recommendations, which are also cited in the Australia and New Zealand position paper on perinatal mental health services.

As I was writing this chapter, Healthscope in Tasmania announced that they would be closing the state's one private mother and baby unit – the only eight beds available. The community was justifiably outraged and a week later the government intervened, announcing plans for a new public MBU at the Royal Hobart Hospital. However, even with the new public unit, there will be fewer beds in the state than before.

Not having access to a nearby MBU will mean that many women fall through the cracks in regional emergency departments not equipped to manage severe perinatal mental illness. This simply isn't good enough.

Non-binary and transgender parents

The experiences of non-binary and transgender birthing parents are only now being recorded and understood.

A 2018 Australian study noted that body changes for trans men were often experienced as 'frightening', 'distressing' and 'difficult to handle', particularly those related to their chests. Said one participant: 'I felt completely in the wrong body, my flesh, the roundness and bulges. The way it felt and looked really frightened me, so foreign, like the more pregnant I got the more alien my skin felt. It terrified me. It wasn't the femaleness of it. It was the intense changes, the physical changes.'

Research into transgender men highlights a lack of education around mental illness in the perinatal period, as well as health professionals lacking knowledge of gender-affirming care and mood – for example, the impact of testosterone. Said one man:

> Healthcare professionals need to know that postpartum depression needs to be talked about more, and it really needs to be talked about with trans men who plan on having babies and plan on breastfeeding, meaning that they won't be getting back on testosterone to level out the hormones. Because that roller coaster was an insanity you cannot describe.

As Edwina Orchard and Sharna Jamadar outline in their paper *Matrescence: Lifetime Impact of Motherhood and Cognition on the Brain*, no study to date has looked at cognitive changes during the journey to parenthood for people whose gender may not match their biological sex. However, as Rosie Charter and Kerry Robinson highlight in their study, many transgender parents felt isolated during the perinatal period, and given isolation is linked to perinatal depression, it's a population likely to be at significant risk.

Perinatal mental health, neurodivergence and parents with a disability

Research is also needed into the perinatal experiences of those who are neurodivergent. This seems particularly urgent given the rise in women being diagnosed with ADHD and/or autism. In 2022, the first study to look at the trajectory of perinatal well-being in autistic people was conducted, finding that they may be more stressed, depressed or anxious than non-autistic people during this period. 'The findings highlight the need for effective screening and support surrounding perinatal well-being for autistic people,' the authors wrote. Understanding and communicating the safety of ADHD medications during pregnancy is also key as diagnoses in women increase.

Two recent studies – one in the United States and one in Canada – found that women with disabilities are at an increased risk of experiencing depressive symptoms during the perinatal period compared to women without disabilities. As the authors of the US study note, women with disabilities also face barriers to receiving equitable care, in addition to 'widespread discriminatory attitudes and biases' of health professionals who question their capacity for pregnancy, birth and parenting.

Such research highlights the importance of adapted screening and inclusive, accessible services for this population of expectant and new parents.

New treatments

As well as existing treatments such as medication, psychotherapy and ECT, new treatments are also emerging. I read about research into the use of ketamine in not just treating PND, but preventing it. Dr Miriam Schultz told *Glamour* in June 2022, 'These studies confirm what I and others see clinically: that ketamine can work on postpartum depression quickly and effectively.'

I watch with interest when the US Food and Drug Administration (FDA) approves Zulresso (brexanolone), the first drug approved specifically for postpartum depression. But while this might sound exciting and promising, it's less so when you read the fine print. It's only available in certain healthcare facilities, requires hospitalisation for sixty hours for the infusion, and costs around US$34,000 (not including in-patient costs). Researchers in the US are currently recruiting participants for a clinical trial to see if Zulresso has the same efficacy on women with postpartum psychosis. The drug hasn't been approved for use in Australia.

In August 2023, the FDA approved Zuranolone, the first oral medication for postpartum depression. One of the benefits of this medication is that it works much faster than other drugs typically prescribed for depression and anxiety – results were seen in just three days. There's still much we don't know, however, and its safety during pregnancy and breastfeeding has yet to be established. Zuranolone also hasn't been approved for use in Australia. (It's important to note, too, that a pill will never be a magic bullet when it comes to treating perinatal mental illness. It's simply one piece of the puzzle.)

In Australia, a team of researchers will soon develop and evaluate an 'ultra-brief' single-session online treatment tailored for women with perinatal depression and anxiety. At a time when affordable care and accessible services remain key barriers to receiving help, it's exciting to see the potential of a quick, low-cost option.

Thanks to Kourtney Kardashian, maternal placentophagy – ingesting your own placenta after birth via everything from placenta pills to placenta smoothies – has also been back in the headlines. Like Chrissy Teigen, who claimed that ingesting her placenta helped ward off postnatal depression, the eldest Kardashian sister shared a picture of her pills on Instagram, noting that they were linked to a 'lesser chance of postpartum depression', among a raft of other 'health benefits'. It's a claim that does the rounds every few years despite the dearth of evidence to support it. In an article for *The Conversation*, 'No, You Shouldn't Eat Your Placenta, Here's Why', Bryony McNeill, a lecturer in reproductive and developmental biology at Deakin University, notes that most of the proposed benefits are based on anecdotal reports from women who have consumed their placentas, and from animal studies. 'We found that there is no scientific evidence of any clinical benefit of placentophagy among humans, and no placental nutrients and hormones are retained in sufficient amounts after placenta encapsulation to be potentially helpful to the mother postpartum.'

Prevention

As early as 1993, in her book *Pregnancy: The Inside Story*, Joan Raphael-Leff noted, 'Unaccountably we have rarely taken prophylactic measures nor exploited preventative opportunities but wait to treat established conditions.'

This is what COPE sought to address through our campaign The Truth and our evidence-based app, underpinned by the national guidelines. Prevention work relies on screening, particularly those identified as high risk, as well as psychoeducation around the emotional and mental challenges of becoming and being a parent. We hear time and again that an expectation gap causes problems for new mums: *This isn't what I was expecting. Why aren't I the mother I thought I'd be?*

But prevention is not without its challenges. Although perinatal mental health issues are common, there's still a belief that 'it won't happen to me'.

At a recent baby expo, a colleague and I manned a COPE stand. Over the weekend, we'd watch as expectant and new parents would walk towards us, see our sign for 'the mental health experts', then bow their heads as if we might be contagious. Many gave us a wide berth and very few came up to ask questions. It was often their parents who'd sidle over, take a flyer and pop it into their bag.

As I write, one of my friends is embarking on a second pregnancy after postpartum psychosis. She is understandably nervous but is working closely with her health team to prepare for all possible outcomes. It's exactly what Emily from Chapter 9 did, too. She recently gave birth to her second baby, a beautiful boy. After a short (planned) stay in the MBU for early monitoring, Emily was discharged home, where she has remained healthy. 'It's a ray of hope for others who might be considering a baby after postpartum psychosis,' she tells me.

As Verinder Sharma and colleagues note, postpartum psychosis should be preventable in some cases because at-risk women can be identified and monitored. Also, we know when the onset period is – symptoms begin or worsen immediately after delivery in most cases, or sometimes begin in late pregnancy – and that it is short and limited to a few weeks (or sometimes months) after delivery.

Professor Buist tells me of research she and her colleagues conducted around sleep deprivation with women who had previous experience of postpartum psychosis. Participants in the study gave birth during the day – either by a C-section or being induced. 'The treating psychiatrists were all managing the sleep deprivation and ensuring it didn't happen,' she says. 'We had so few people relapse postpartum. I'm firmly convinced that sleep is a big trigger for at-risk populations. We knew they all had a previous post-partum psychosis, so we knew the next baby was going to be a problem. But we did really well.'

Looking to the future

Born in 2011, Henry belongs to Gen Z. His generation is not only more comfortable talking about mental health, but also more likely to seek professional assistance for mental illness. They're also more likely to be on TikTok, a platform where parents are more inclined to share the less pretty aspects of pregnancy, motherhood and parenthood than their millennial counterparts on Instagram. (I once saw a TikTok of a young mum pointing to facts about intrusive thoughts in the perinatal period while the viral song 'Happiness' played. Watching it was like an out-of-body experience and made me realise I am, in fact, approaching middle age.)

Research shows that Gen Z portray themselves as a 'generation of contrasts: powerful and self-assured, yet vulnerable and damaged'. They're also more likely to opt out of parenthood entirely, with many citing the climate crisis and the cost of living as reasons for not having children or for having fewer children than they otherwise wanted.

Speaking to colleagues at conferences around Australia recently, I've felt a growing sense of excitement and optimism in the field of perinatal mental health. We're also now seeing sub-specialities evolving, such as those focusing on birth trauma or on supporting the needs of couples. But experience and knowledge are pieces of a bigger puzzle, and a collaborative, interconnected approach is required. This is particularly the case in a sector where many organisations compete for state and federal funding and where programs rely on continued support. 'There's no point recommending services or apps if they're not going to be around in six months,' one midwife told me at a conference recently.

I ask Nicole for her thoughts on where perinatal mental health currently stands in Australia. 'We have learned so much in the evolution of perinatal mental health,' she says. 'And while gaps in the evidence remain to be explored and understood, innovation is providing with us ever more opportunities to embed elements of best practice in a way that is sustainable, inclusive and measurable.'

When it comes to priority areas, Nicole agrees that Australia needs more mother and baby units – and not just in metropolitan locations. Improving screening rates in the private health system is also key, as is continuing to build the workforce so that women receive evidence-based care when they're referred for treatment. There's also a need for more education about safe use of medications during pregnancy and breastfeeding as well as a focus on screening dads and non-birthing partners.

'There's always more work to do,' she says. 'But it's an exciting time to be doing it – and I'm glad you're doing it with us.'

The Facts

- Up to 80 per cent of women will experience the baby blues. This usually occurs around day three to five and coincides with hormonal changes happening post-birth.
- In Australia, perinatal depression and anxiety affects one in five mothers.
- Up to one in ten fathers experience depression between the first trimester and one year postpartum.
- Severe depression during the perinatal period is associated with maternal suicide.
- Postpartum psychosis occurs in 1-2 in 1000 pregnancies. It is a psychiatric emergency, but it is highly treatable.
- One in three Australian women experience their birth as being traumatic. Partners and non-birthing parents can also experience birth trauma.
- Perinatal OCD rates vary between approximately 8 and 17 per cent.

Helplines and Support

Australian Breastfeeding Association
A national 24/7 breastfeeding helpline – 1800 686 268
www.breastfeeding.asn.au

Australasian Birth Trauma Association
A peer-led community dedicated to helping Australians and
New Zealanders prevent and heal from birth-related trauma.
https://birthtrauma.org.au

Butterfly Foundation
A national charity providing support for body image issues
and eating disorders.
https://butterfly.org.au

Beyond PP Facebook Group
A Facebook community for those in Australia and New Zealand
who've experienced postpartum psychosis.
https://www.facebook.com/groups/473249929541274

Centre of Perinatal Excellence (COPE)
A not-for-profit organisation devoted to reducing the impacts
of emotional and mental health problems in the pre- and
postnatal periods.
https://cope.org.au

eCOPE Directory – A national database of clinicians with expertise in perinatal mental health and community support services.
https://directory.cope.org.au

Ready to COPE app – A free app that prepares new and expectant parents for the emotional and mental challenges of becoming and being a parent.
https://www.cope.org.au/readytocope

Circle of Security
Resources for parents and professionals from the Circle of Security program.
https://www.circleofsecurityinternational.com

ForWhen
A national support line connecting parents to the right service during pregnancy and postpartum – 1300 24 23 22
https://forwhenhelpline.org.au

Gidget Foundation Australia
Gidget Foundation Australia provides free face-to-face individual psychological counselling sessions for expectant and new parents, as well as telehealth via Start Talking.
https://www.gidgetfoundation.org.au

Lifeline
A national charity providing 24-hour crisis support and suicide prevention services – 13 11 14
https://www.lifeline.org.au

PANDA (Perinatal Depression & Anxiety Australia)
National perinatal mental health helpline – 1300 726 306
https://panda.org.au

Acknowledgements

Reading the acknowledgments of books has always been one of my favourite pastimes – seeing the support, labour, encouragement and love that sits behind their creation. It takes a village to raise a child (they say) and it has taken a village to write this memoir.

Thank you for your help and advice in the early stages of this project when it was just a collection of notes and a long-held dream: Andrew Pippos, Tim Douglas, Kylie Orr, Rochelle Siemienowicz, Léa Antigny, Anna Spargo-Ryan, Aaron Richards, Lucinda Beaman, Kate Aubusson, Matthew Broome, Guy Longworth, Matt Haig, John Purcell, Kon Karapanagiotidis and Jenny Valentish.

Thank you, Natalie Reilly, for publishing 'The Year My Brain Broke' and making me realise there was a book there and that I needed to write it. Here it is, Nat!

To my agent, Benython Oldfield, for believing in this book from day one and making sure it found the perfect home. Thank you also to Sharon for being such a great supporter and for kind and insightful feedback.

To my publisher, Sophy Williams at Black Inc., who appeared in a beam of light on Zoom the first time we met and has been a beam of light since. You knew exactly what I wanted to achieve with this book – thank you for making my dream come true and for recognising how important this issue is.

To my editors, Jo Rosenberg and Rebecca Bauert: as soon as I met you both, I knew I'd be in good hands. You have shown me so much kindness, patience and grace and have made this book infinitely better. How lucky I've been.

Thank you, Alissa Dinallo, for such a beautiful cover. I still can't stop looking at it.

Thank you to Caitlin Yates, Elisabeth Young, Kate Nash, Aira Pimping and everyone working behind the scenes at Black Inc. This experience has been so much fun and such a pleasure and I'm so grateful.

Thank you to my wonderful friends who've held me both literally and from afar when writing this has been difficult. Thank you in particular to Darren Saunders, Eddie, Marc, Kylie, Heidi Krause, Bek Omond, Lauren Dickinson, Carly-Jay Metcalfe and Charlie Faulder. Thank you also to the lovely Debut Crew of fellow authors releasing their firstborns into the world this year. The support, camaraderie, humour and wisdom has been a heart-lift.

To Paul Filipczyk – for teaching me how to do good, solid work with heart and integrity. Thank you for the knotty, difficult conversations that made this book better.

Lizzie – I am who I am in part because we met all those years ago. You brought me out of my shell with your colour and chaos and kindness and loyalty. Doing this life by your side is a privilege and a treat.

Paul G. – I'm so glad our paths crossed all those years ago as baby psychs. You are a force. My world is better for having you in it.

To Chloe Angyal, whose book *Turning Pointe* and writing on ballet has helped me understand my own complicated feelings around dance. Thank you for giving me the language and critical thought to help make it better for the next generation of dancers.

Thank you to those who looked at very undercooked earlier

drafts with kindness and excellent ideas – Luke Carman, Marty McKenzie-Murray and GW. (Thank you, GW, for the conversation that clarified everything.)

To Camila Gonzalez Martinez – thank you for your kind edits, insightful suggestions and for being such a hype girl. What a joy you are – how lucky this industry is to have you.

Thank you, Susan Johnson, whose own memoir *A Better Woman* made me realise it was possible to write a memoir about motherhood with candour, humour and my whole damn heart.

To my former child protection colleagues, in particular DC, Michelle Sopuch and Alison Soutter.

To the mothers I met on the MBU, especially you, dear M and beautiful Carolyn (and Si). To finding friendship in the lowest of places.

To the 'Brookes' who tried to help – thank you and I'm sorry.

To Emma Pollard – I'll never forget how you showed up.

To my boss and mentor, Nicole Highet. Thank you for opening the door to perinatal mental health when I was a little lost and not sure what was supposed to come next. I know what comes next now and I'm so pleased to be doing it beside you. Thank you to the COPE team, who are the most passionate and inspiring group of people. I'm so proud of what we've achieved.

Thank you to Professor Anne Buist for being so generous with your time and expertise.

To Olivia Jenkins, who helped me fall in love with ballet again, and Elena Lambrinos, who took a chance on a novice who needed to unlearn ballet to be able to teach it. Dance has kept me (relatively) sane while writing this book. I'm glad it found me again.

Thank you to Emily, Rebecca and Melinda for sharing your stories with me and with the world. As my colleague Michael said, 'It is no small thing, being so honest.'

To the childcare workers at SDN Redfern (in particular Simita, Rochelle, Aunty Trish and Doris) who cared for Henry from the time before he could walk until he started primary school. You wrapped around our little family when we needed it most and we will never forget your kindness and generosity.

To the women of the Beyond PP Facebook group, who have been so candid with their thoughts, advice and recollections around postpartum psychosis and are some of the strongest, fiercest women I've met.

To Cheri Wissmann and Willemijn de Bruin of the PPP Awareness Day team. Thank you for introducing me to other women around the world who are doing advocacy work for perinatal psychosis and for clarifying and insightful conversations around aspects of PP treatment.

Lucy Ormonde, you published my very first article at *Mamamia* and made me believe I might be able to write. Thank you.

Thank you to Amber Robinson, Melanie Mahoney and Katie Carlin of *Essential Baby* for helping me build a new career when I was floundering. So many elements of this book grew out of pieces you commissioned and published.

To Mum and Dad. Thank you for always supporting me – in dance, in writing, in my career and in life. I love you both so much. Thank you for the poetry, Mum, for your astute, insightful edits and for picking up every single missing word, stray comma and not-so-elegant phrase in this manuscript. (I've had so many people ask, 'Can she please do mine next?') And thank you, Dad, for passing on the driest humour, the deepest empathy and endless curiosity.

To my beautiful Nonna, who at ninety-seven is still singing, reading and doing yoga. You always knew I'd write this book. This book is also for you. To my aunts, Glyn and Meri, for your love and support always, but particularly while I was so unwell.

To my siblings, Evan, Lulu and Huw. I am so lucky to have the three of you, my beautiful nieces and nephews and brother-in-law, Pete. Evan, you stepped in and kept stepping in for me but also for Henry. How to articulate the depth of my gratitude? Thank you.

Amy, how lucky I am that you married my brother. Thank you for your kindness, intelligence and for remembering some funny (and not-so-funny) things I'd completely forgotten.

To the Beestons – Penny, Rob, Jacqui and Milly, and my brother-in-law, Nick Lukowski. I've been part of your family since day one, wrapped in love and unconditional support. Thank you, Penny, for your kind feedback on an early draft and for always encouraging my writing. Best mother-in-law I've ever had – I don't expect to do any better in future.

To Dr Q, I wouldn't be here without you. Thank you for holding me and for saving me both postpartum and while re-living these postpartum years. You put me back together again when I thought I was too broken to fix. I like to think I'm some of your best work. If I wasn't too medicated to cry, I'd cry.

To my boys – Robb and Hen. When I filed my very messy first draft, the feedback (from everyone) was 'more Robb'. Who could blame them? I'll always want 'more Robb' too. Thank you for being my sounding-board, my compass, my partner in life and my biggest cheerleader. Going back over such painful memories (again and again and again) has been harrowing at times and I'm so grateful for your patience, bravery and humour. I wouldn't have made it without you.

Hen, you are my joy and my heart and my heart and my joy.

This book is my love letter to you both. Thank you, thank you, thank you. I love you, I love you, I love you.

References and Further Reading

1. Level One
Tony Kushner, *Angels in America: A Gay Fantasia on National Themes*, Theatre Communications Group, New York, 1996.

3. Rorschach Test
Anne Carson, 'The Glass Essay', *Glass, Irony and God*, New Directions Publishing Corporation, 1995.
M. Davis, *Family Is Culture Review*, Report, Independent Review of Aboriginal Children and Young People in Out of Home Care (OOHC), NSW Government, Sydney, 2019.
Sharon Lamb, *The Not Good Enough Mother*, Beacon Press, Boston, 2019.
Sarah Sentilles, *Stranger Care: A Memoir of Loving What Isn't Ours*, Text Publishing, Melbourne, 2021.
Maggie Smith, *You Could Make This Place Beautiful*, Simon & Schuster, New York, 2022.
Elizabeth Wall-Wieler et al., 'Maternal Mental Health After Custody Loss and Death of a Child: A Retrospective Cohort Study Using Linkable Administrative Data', *Canadian Journal of Psychiatry*, vol. 63, 2018, pp. 322–8.

4. The Spark That Fires the Mind
Patricia A. Brennan et al., 'Maternal Depression and Infant Cortisol: Influences of Timing, Comorbidity and Treatment', *Journal of*

Child Psychology and Psychiatry, vol. 49, no. 10, Oct 2008, pp. 1099–107.

Heather Christle, *The Crying Book*, Catapult, New York, 2019.

Joan Didion, *The Year of Magical Thinking*, Knopf, New York, 2006.

N.J. Highet and the Expert Working Group and Expert Subcommittees, *Mental Health Care in the Perinatal Period: Australian Clinical Practice Guideline*, Centre of Perinatal Excellence, Melbourne, 2023.

Gelsey Kirkland with Greg Lawrence, *Dancing On My Grave*, Doubleday, New York, 1986.

Leslie Jamison, 'The Quickening', *The Atlantic*, September 2019.

J.W. Palmer, *Puerperal Insanity*, address to Georgia Medical Association, 1903, https://www.ncbi.nlm.nih.gov/pmc/articles/PMC8953002/pdf/atlantajrecmed141958-0005.pdf.

Pedestrian TV, 'Top Five Post Baby Body Bounce Backs', *Pedestrian*, 2011.

Alana Rogers et al., 'Association Between Maternal Perinatal Depression and Anxiety and Child and Adolescent Development: A Meta-analysis', *JAMA Pediatrics*, vol. 174, no. 11, 2020, pp. 1082–92.

Brittany Watson et al., 'The Meaning of Body Image Experiences During the Perinatal Period: A Systematic Review of the Qualitative Literature', *Body Image*, vol. 14, 2015, pp. 102–13.

5. The Republic of Motherhood

Margaret Atwood, *Dancing Girls and Other Stories*, McClelland and Stewart, Toronto, 1977.

Susan Johnson, *A Better Woman*, Washington Square Press, New York, 1999.

Liz Berry, *The Republic of Motherhood*, Random House, 2018.

Gwen Harwood, 'Mother, Who Gave Me Life', in *The Lion's Bride: Selected Poetry*, Angus and Robertson, Sydney, 1981, pp. 75–76.

Catherine Pierce, 'How Becoming a Mother Is Like Space Travel', in *Danger Days*, Saturnalia Books, 2020.

Sylvia Plath, 'Morning Song', in *Collected Poems*, HarperCollins, 1960.

Dana Raphael, *Being Female: Reproduction, Power, and Change*, De Gruyter Mouton, New York, 1975.

The Royal Australian and New Zealand College of Obstetricians and Gynaecologists, *Instrumental Vaginal Birth*, March 2020.

K.M. Robson and R. Kumar, 'Delayed Onset of Maternal Affection After Childbirth', *The British Journal of Psychiatry*, vol. 136, no. 4, 1980, pp. 347–53.

Idun Røseth et al., 'New Mothers' Struggles to Love Their Child. An Interpretative Synthesis of Qualitative Studies', *International Journal of Qualitative Studies on Health and Well-being*, vol. 13, no. 1, December 2018.

Jelena Stojanov et al., 'Postpartum Psychiatric Disorders: Review of the Research History, Classification, Epidemiological Data, Etiological Factors and Clinical Presentations', *Acta Facultatis Medicae Naissensis*, vol. 36, 2019, pp. 167–76.

Sue White et al., *Reassessing Attachment Theory in Child Welfare*, Bristol University Press, 2019.

6. Lactation Madness

Robert Frost, 'Stopping by Woods on a Snowy Evening', *The Poetry of Robert Frost*, ed. Edward Connery Lathem, Henry Holt & Co., New York, 1969.

Charlotte Perkins Gillman, 'The Yellow Wallpaper', first published in *The New English Magazine*, 1892.

Maggie Nelson, *The Argonauts*, Graywolf Press, Minneapolis, 2015.

Tore Nielsen and Tyna Paquette, 'Dream-Associated Behaviors Affecting Pregnant and Postpartum Women', *Sleep*, vol. 30, no. 9, September 2007, pp. 1162–9.

Nancy Williams, 'Maternal Psychological Issues in the Experience of Breastfeeding', *Journal of Human Lactation*, vol. 13, no. 1, 1997, pp. 57–60.

7. Dragon Baby

Marie-Paule Austin, 'Postpartum Psychosis: A Practical Management Guide for Obstetricians,' *O&G Magazine*, vol. 20, no. 3, Spring 2018.

Pam Belluck, 'After Baby an Unravelling', *The New York Times*, 16 June 2014.

M. Galbally et al., 'Comparison of Public Mother–Baby Psychiatric Units in Australia: Similarities, Strengths and Recommendations', *Australasian Psychiatry*, vol. 27, no. 2, 2019, pp. 112–16.

Rivka Galchen, *Little Labors*, New Directions, New York, 2016.

Usham S. Neill, 'Tom Cruise Is Dangerous and Irresponsible', *Journal of Clinical Investigation*, vol. 115, no. 8, August 2005, pp. 1964–5.

Brooke Shields, 'War of Words', *The New York Times*, 1 July 2005.

Rachel Yoder, *Nightbitch*, Penguin Random House, New York, 2022.

8. If They Make Me Do Art Therapy

Mary D. Salter Ainsworth et al., *Patterns of Attachment: A Psychological Study of the Strange Situation*, Lawrence Erlbaum, New York, 1978.

Mary D. Salter Ainsworth and Silvia M. Bell, 'Attachment, Exploration, and Separation: Illustrated by the Behaviour of One-Year-Olds in a Strange Situation', *Child Development*, vol. 41, 1970, pp. 49–67.

C. Evans, J. Kreppner and P.J. Lawrence, 'The Association Between Maternal Perinatal Mental Health and Perfectionism: A Systematic Review and Meta-Analysis', *British Journal of Clinical Psychology*, vol. 61, no. 4, 28 June 2022, pp. 1052–74.

Nichole Fairbrother et al., 'Postpartum Thoughts of Infant-Related Harm and Obsessive-Compulsive Disorder: Relation to Maternal Physical Aggression Toward the Infant', *Journal of Clinical Psychiatry*, vol. 83, no. 2, 1 March 2022.

Pehr Granqvist et al., 'Disorganized Attachment in Infancy: A Review of the Phenomenon and Its Implications for Clinicians and Policy-Makers', *Attachment and Human Development*, vol. 19, no. 6, 2017, pp. 534–58.

Kay Redfield Jamison, *An Unquiet Mind: A Memoir of Moods and Madness*, Knopf, New York, 1995.

Susan Sontag, 'Dancer and the Dance', *London Review of Books*, 5 February 1987.

E. Tronick et al., 'Infant Emotions in Normal and Pertubated Interactions', paper presented at the biennial meeting of the Society for Research in Child Development, Denver, C.O., April 1975.

Sarah E. Victor et al., 'Only Human: Mental-Health Difficulties Among Clinical, Counseling, and School Psychology Faculty and Trainees', *Perspectives on Psychological Science*, vol. 17, no. 6, November 2022, pp. 1576–90.

D.W. Winnicott, 'Transitional Object and Transitional Phenomena', *International Journal of Psychoanalysis*, vol. 34, 1953, pp. 89–97.

Fiona Wright, *Small Acts of Disappearance: Essays on Hunger*, Giramondo, Penrith, 2015.

9. What Goes Up

Diana Jefferies et al., 'The River of Postnatal Psychosis: A Qualitative Study of Women's Experiences and Meanings', *Midwifery*, December 2021.

Katherine McEvoy, 'Clinical Phenotypes of Postpartum Psychosis', in Jennifer L. Payne and Lauren M. Osborne, *Biomarkers of Postpartum Psychiatric Disorders*, Academic Press, Johns Hopkins University, 2020, pp. 137–47.

The Lancet Psychiatry, 'Post-partum Psychosis: Birth of a New Disorder?', *The Lancet*, vol. 8, no. 12, December 2021.

Margaret Spinelli, 'Postpartum Psychosis: A Diagnosis for the DSMV', *Archives of Women's Mental Health*, vol. 24, 2021, pp. 817–22.

Rachel VanderKruik et al., 'The Global Prevalence of Postpartum Psychosis: A Systematic Review', *BMC Psychiatry*, vol. 17, no. 1, 28 July 2017, p. 272.

10. I Don't Think These Hands Are Mine

Irivin Yalom, *Staring at the Sun*, Scribe Publications, Melbourne, 2008.

Vladimir Nabokov, *Speak, Memory: An Autobiography Revisited*, Putnam, New York, 1966.

11. How Did the Baby Live?

Australia's Mothers and Babies, web report, Australian Institute of Health and Welfare, Canberra, 2022. Available at www.aihw.gov.au/reports/mothers-babies/australias-mothers-babies/contents/maternal-deaths.

DPP v MA [2022] VSC 170, 7 April 2022.

DPP v Nguyen [2023] VSC 325, 14 June 2023.

Karen Kleiman, *Therapy and the Postpartum Woman: Notes on Healing Postpartum Depression for Clinicians and the Women Who Seek their Help*, Routledge, London, 2008.

Faith McLellan, 'Mental Health and Justice: The Case of Andrea Yates', *The Lancet*, vol. 368, no. 9551, 2 December 2006, pp. 1951–54.

Louis-Victor Marcé, *Treatise on Insanity in Pregnant, Postpartum and Lactating Women*, Baillière, Paris, 1858.

Margaret Oates, 'Suicide: The Leading Cause of Maternal Death', *The British Journal of Psychiatry*, vol. 183, no. 4, October 2003, pp. 279–81.

R v Seville (a pseudonym) [2023] NSWSC 556, 25 May 2023.

Charlene Thornton et al., 'Maternal Deaths in NSW (2000–2006) from Nonmedical Causes (Suicide and Trauma) in the First Year Following Birth', *BioMed Research International*, 2013.

12. Transference

Jonathan Shedler, 'That Was Then, This Is Now: Psychoanalytic Psychotherapy for the Rest of Us', *Contemporary Psychoanalysis*, vol. 58, no. 2–3, 2022, pp. 405–37.

14. Real Isn't How You're Made

Nuar Alsadir, *Animal Joy*, Fitzcarraldo Editions, London, 2022.

Vaughan Bell and Jorge Carlos Holguín-Lew, 'When I Want to Cry I Can't. Inability to Cry Following SSRI Treatment', *Revista Colombiana de Psiquiatría*, December 2013, pp. 304–10.

Gabrielle Calvocoressi, 'At Last the New Arriving,' in *Apocalyptic Swing*, Persea Books, New York, 2009.

Karen Kleiman, 'Holding Perinatal Women in Distress', *Psychology Today*, 9 February 2017.

D.W. Winnicott, 'Ego Distortion in Terms of True and False Self', in *The Maturational Processes and the Facilitating Environment*, International Universities Press, New York, 1965, pp. 140–52.

Margery Williams, *The Velveteen Rabbit*, George H. Doran Company, Toronto, 1922.

Jeanette Winterson, *Why Be Happy When You Could Be Normal?*, Grove Press, London, 2013.

15. There Are Three People in My Marriage

Ariane Beeston, 'There Are Three People in My Marriage', *Mamamia*, 15 July 2013.

Nora Ephron, *Heartburn*, Alfred A. Knopf, New York, 1983.

Benedicte Johannsen et al., 'Divorce or Separation Following Postpartum Psychiatric Episodes: A Population-Based Cohort Study', *The Journal of Clinical Psychiatry*, 23 March 2021.

16. I Hold My Breath Until My Breath Holds Me

'Postpartum Psychosis', Royal College of Psychiatrists, 2018.

17. The Year My Brain Broke

Ariane Beeston, 'The Year My Brain Broke', *The Sydney Morning Herald*, 15 February 2018.

E.N. Bider and J.L. Coker, 'Postpartum Psychosis and SARS-Cov-2 Infection: Is There a Correlation?', *Archive of Women's Health*, vol. 24, no. 6, December 2021, pp. 1051–54.

N.J. Highet and C.A. Purtell, 'The National Perinatal Depression Initiative: A Synopsis of Progress to Date and Recommendations for Beyond 2013', Beyond Blue, August 2012.

A.A. Subramanyam et al., 'Postpartum Psychosis in Mothers with SARS-CoV-2 Infection: A Case Series from India', *Asian Journal of Psychiatry*, 2020.

Adrienne Rich, *On Lies, Secrets and Silence: Selected Prose*, W.W. Norton & Company, New York, 1979.

18. Well, What Do You Expect?

Deborah Levy, *Things I Don't Want to Know*, Penguin, London, 2018.

20. I'm Just So Glad I'm Here

Sean Thomas Dougherty, 'Why Bother?', *The Second O of Sorrow*, BOA Editions, Rochester, N.Y., 2018.

Martha Graham, 'Martha Graham Reflects on Her Art and Life in Dance', *The New York Times*, 31 March 1985.

Elaine Graser, 'Parent Trap: Why the Cult of the Perfect Mother Has to End', *The Guardian*, 18 May 2021.

Zelda Grimshaw, 'Mothering: Feminism's Unfinished Business', *The Age*, 1 August 2002.

Karen Kleiman, *The Art of Holding in Therapy: An Essential Intervention for Postpartum Depression and Anxiety*, Routledge, London, 2018.

Emily Leibert, 'Hidden Pain, Controlled Bodies: Does Ballet Have to Be Like This?', *Jezebel*, 12 June 2023.

Ann Oakley, *Women Confined: Towards a Sociology of Childbirth*, Schocken Books, New York, 1980.

Adrienne Rich, *Of Woman Born: Motherhood as Experience and Institution*, W.W. Norton & Co., New York, 1976.

Andrew Solomon, 'Grieving for the Therapist Who Taught Me How to Grieve,' *The New Yorker*, 10 May 2020.

Natalie Stevens, Nicole Heath, Teresa Lillis et al., 'Examining the Effectiveness of a Coordinated Perinatal Mental Health Care Model Using an Intersectional-feminist Perspective', *Journal of Behavioral Medicine*, vol. 41, no. 5, October 2018, pp. 627–40.

Erin Vincent, 'They Say Writing Is Cathartic But Writing My Memoir Almost Killed Me', *The Guardian*, 11 April 2017.

Appendix

Births, Australia, 2022, Australian Bureau of Statistics, 18 October 2023.

Anneli Andersson et al., 'Depression and Anxiety Disorders During the Postpartum Period in Women Diagnosed with Attention

Deficit Hyperactivity Disorder', *Journal of Affective Disorders*, vol. 15, no. 325, March 2023, pp. 817–23.

Jeanne L. Alhusen et al., 'Depressive Symptoms During the Perinatal Period by Disability Status: Findings from the United States Pregnancy Risk Assessment Monitoring System', *Journal of Advanced Nursing*, vol. 79, no. 1, January 2023, pp. 223–33.

Hilary Brown et al., 'Perinatal Mental Illness Among Women with Disabilities: A Population-Based Cohort Study', *Social Psychiatry and Psychiatric Epidemiology*, vol. 57, no. 11, November 2022, pp. 2217–28.

Anne Buist et al., 'Mother-Baby Psychiatric Units in Australia – The Victorian Experience', *Archives of Women's Mental Health*, vol. 7, no. 1, February 2004, pp. 81–7.

C. Chamberlain et al., 'Supporting Aboriginal and Torres Strait Islander Families to Stay Together from the Start (Safest Start): Urgent Call to Action to Address Crisis in Infant Removals', *Australian Journal of Social Issues*, vol. 57, no. 2, 2022, pp. 252–73.

Daria Daehn et al., 'Perinatal Mental Health Literacy: Knowledge, Attitudes, and Help-Seeking Among Perinatal Women and the Public – A Systematic Review', *BMC Pregnancy Childbirth*, vol. 22, no. 574, 2022.

K.M. Deligiannidis et al., 'Zuranolone for the Treatment of Postpartum Depression', *American Journal of Psychiatry*, vol. 180, no. 9, 1 September 2023, pp. 668–75.

Fairbrother N. et al., 'High Prevalence and Incidence of Obsessive-Compulsive Disorder Among Women Across Pregnancy and the Postpartum', *Journal of Clinical Psychiatry*, vol. 82, no. 2, 23 March 2021.

E.J. Ford et al., 'Pregnancy Risk Factors Associated with Birthweight of Infants Born to Australian Aboriginal Women in an Urban Setting – A Retrospective Cohort Study', *BMC Pregnancy Childbirth*, vol. 18, no. 382, 2018.

Sarah Hampton et al., 'Autistic Mothers' Perinatal Well-Being and Parenting Styles', *Autism*, vol. 26, no. 7, 2022.

Alexis Hoffkling, Juno Obedin-Maliver and Jae Sevelius, 'From Erasure to Opportunity: A Qualitative Study of the Experiences of Transgender Men Around Pregnancy and Recommendations for Providers', *BMC Pregnancy Childbirth*, vol. 17 (Suppl 2), no. 332, 8 November 2017.

Katrina Moss et al., 'How Rates of Perinatal Mental Health Screening in Australia Have Changed Over Time and Which Women Are Missing Out', *Australian and New Zealand Journal of Public Health*, 8 June 2020.

Edwina Orchard et al., 'Matrescence: Lifetime Impact of Motherhood on Cognition and the Brain', *Trends in Cognitive Science*, 27 March 2023.

'The Cost of PNDA in Australia', Gidget Foundation Australia, 2019.

'Perinatal Mental Health Services', Position Statement, The Royal Australian and New Zealand College of Psychiatrists, October 2021.

Joan Raphael-Leff, *Pregnancy: The Inside Story*, Routledge, London, 1993.

Nicole Reilly et al., 'Disparities in Reported Psychosocial Assessment Across Public and Private Maternity Settings: A National Survey of Women in Australia', *BMC Public Health*, vol. 13, no. 632, 4 July 2013.

Verinder Sharma et al., 'Postpartum Psychosis: Revisiting the Phenomenology, Nosology, and Treatment', *Journal of Affective Disorders Reports*, vol. 10, 2022.

Sarah Wynter, 'Sarah Wynter Suffered Postpartum Psychosis. She Survived to Make a Movie About It', *Vanity Fair*, January 2022.